Essential Oils
for EMOTIONAL WELLBEING

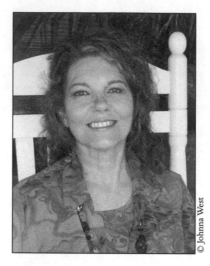

About the Author

Vannoy Gentles Fite is the author of *Essential Oils for Healing* and currently lives in Saltillo, Texas. Fite has two beautiful daughters, one wonderful stepdaughter, three grandsons, and two granddaughters. Fite is a certified Ayurvedic lifestyle coach, a certified herbalist, a licensed yoga instructor, and a certified aromatherapist. She believes wholeheartedly in natural healing methods, yoga, Ayurveda, and living mindfully and sustainably. She lives her life as spiritually as her path allows and is forever growing as a soul. Fite continues to grow her own vegetable garden and herbs, instructs and practices yoga, raises chickens, ducks, and fish, studies Ayurveda, and is a part of a family of crazy misfits and unique individuals.

EM: vannoylou@gmail.com

FB: Vannoy Gentles Fite, Author

IG: @vannoylou

Amazon: www.amazon.com/author/vannoyfite

Goodreads: www.goodreads.com/goodreadscomauthor/vannoyfite

Essential Oils

for EMOTIONAL WELLBEING

More Than 400 Aromatherapy Recipes for
Mind, Emotions & Spirit

VANNOY GENTLES FITE

Llewellyn Publications
Woodbury, Minnesota

FIRST EDITION
First Printing, 2018

Cover design by Kristi Carlson
Editing by Brian R. Erdrich

Llewellyn Publications is a registered trademark of Llewellyn Worldwide Ltd.

Library of Congress Cataloging-in-Publication Data
    Names: Fite, Vannoy Gentles, author.
    Title: Essential oils for emotional wellbeing : more than 400 aromatherapy
      recipes for mind, emotions & spirit / Vannoy Gentles Fite.
    Description: First edition. | Woodbury, Minnesota : Llewellyn Publications,
      [2018] | Includes bibliographical references and index.
    Identifiers: LCCN 2018028679 (print) | LCCN 2018029595 (ebook) | ISBN
      9780738756721 (ebook) | ISBN 9780738756639 (alk. paper)
    Subjects: LCSH: Essences and essential oils--Therapeutic use. | Mental
      health--Treatment.
    Classification: LCC RM666.A68 (ebook) | LCC RM666.A68 F577 2018 (print) | DDC
      615.3/219—dc23
    LC record available at https://lccn.loc.gov/2018028679

Llewellyn Publications
A Division of Llewellyn Worldwide Ltd.
2143 Wooddale Drive
Woodbury, MN 55125-2989
www.llewellyn.com

Printed in the United States of America

Other books by Vannoy Gentles Fite

Essential Oils for Healing

My parents,
Thomas N. Gentles and Vannoy K. Gentles

Disclaimer

Using essential oils can be very rewarding as long as certain precautions are taken. Simple steps can ensure you have a safe and enjoyable lifetime of usage from your oils. Heed the warnings about each oil in this book and their interactions with medications. If you have any medical conditions, your physician can work with you to ensure that your safety when using essential oils is paramount. I am in no way qualified as a doctor or a diagnostician and cannot condone using essential oils for any ailment without your doctor's express permission.

Contents

Chapter 4: RECIPES FOR EMOTIONS   145

Recipe List

This list includes all of the 400+ recipes that are included in this book. The various recipe methods are listed (bath bomb, lip balm, lotion, etc.), and under each method are all of the recipes that used that method. In parenthesis after each recipe title is the condition, emotion, need, desire, or devotion that the recipe was used for and is listed under in this book. This is a great browsing feature that enables you to scan over 400 recipe titles in minutes.

Bath Recipes

Bath and Shower Bomb Recipes

Bath Salt Recipes

Compress Recipes

Diffuser Recipes

Lip Balm Recipes

Lotion Recipes

Massage Oil Recipes

Neat Recipes

Ointment Recipes

Roller Bottle Recipes

Rub Recipes

Spritzer Recipes

Sugar Scrub Recipes

Wrap Recipes

Introduction

*C*oming from a family of high-strung, addictive, compulsive, and emotionally wounded members, I have thought, studied, and researched mood-enhancing and emotional healing methods all of my life. Learning how to cope with and eradicate certain negative influences and to promote positivity has been at the forefront of my brain since I was a young girl. Studying natural versus pharmaceutical healing is a lifelong passion of mine.

Essential oils have proven to be the answer to my quest. I can use these without anyone even being aware that I am protecting myself from their negative moods or that I am changing their outlooks on the day with a dose of positive oils in the air. I can take myself from a lethargic couch potato to an efficient multitasker in five minutes flat with a dose of these mood-enhancing beauties. Essential oils can have so many beneficial effects on every aspect of our daily lives and on the lives of those around us. This book shows you how to use essential oils for the mind, emotions, and soul.

My first book, *Essential Oils for Healing,* focused on healing everyday ailments with essential oils. *Essential Oils for Emotional Well-Being* is about nurturing those emotional, spiritual, and mental needs that we all have. We are constantly searching for ways to heal ourselves and those around us. Using natural healing techniques can profoundly affect our mental and physical health without causing further harm, which is often not the case with pharmaceuticals. Learning how essential oils can actually have a physical effect on the different areas of the brain, how molecules from the oils can cross that blood/brain barrier, has always been fascinating to me. The fact that by simply smelling an oil can alter how we think or feel is totally mind-blowing when you think about it. But it's true.

I have spent over twenty years researching the emotional effects of essential oils on mental, emotional, and spiritual needs and deficits, and I have incorporated the best blends and recipes in this book for you. Through discussions and work with licensed clinical aromatherapists, certified Ayurvedic practitioners, and certified aromatherapists (I am certified in both Ayurvedic healing and aromatherapy), we have developed, experimented with, and researched the recipes included in this book.

I have previously published a book, *Essential Oils for Healing,* that delves into the physical aspects of healing with essential oils. I have sold essential oils, blends, and recipes for over a decade. I am an essential oil consultant and researcher by profession. My life has been devoted to the study and safe usage of essential oils, and developing this book has been at the forefront of my life for over four years. I truly believe that my higher power gave me both emotions and every plant on earth to use to control those emotions.

This book has been a joy, a learning experience, and a balm to my soul throughout the whole process. The recipes that you use with yourself or your family will be memory-enhancing aromas that, for the rest of your lives, you will associate with healing, positivity, and life enhancement. I pray you have many years of good use from this book and that some of these recipes become as dear to you and your family's heart as they are to mine.

History of Essential Oils

Essential oil history is complex, vast, and spans the world. The different ways that people have used essential oils throughout history is intriguing and sometimes unbelievable. Essential oils are mentioned over one hundred times in the Christian Bible. Our ancestors were extremely awe-inspiring in the ways they incorporated essential oils into not just healing and saving lives, but in every aspect of their daily routines and healing methods. Herbs, plants, and the oils derived from them were the main components of healing in every culture on earth for hundreds of thousands of years.

The usage of essential oils has been found by anthropologists to date as far back as 2800 BC, and some cave drawings suggest that the plants and herbs were turned into oils thousands of years before that. People used the oils as a way to protect themselves from insects, as aromatics, and for culinary uses.

The first people to document the way that they used essential oils in healing were in Egypt and the Middle East. They used the oils for aromatics and eventually discovered that the oils led to healing and even changed emotions when used at various times. The oils were often forbidden to the poorer people and mainly used by royalty and the upper classes. Doctors of ancient times were eventually allowed to treat people with the oils, and their healing benefits quickly spread throughout the world.

One of the most widely known instances in the history of essential oils was the embalming of the deceased by Egyptians using cedar and myrrh essential oil. They incorporated essential oils with various ingredients to mummify their dead, and some of those embalmed mummies are intact today, thousands of years later.

Trade routes were developed in Egypt and the Middle East to carry, sell, and spread the essential oils to various cultures, cities, and countries. Great cities around the world today were developed on these trade routes, and their economic commerce depended on the availability of the plants and trees from which the oils were made.

Ancient scholars used the oils in treating and healing the sick, and taught others to use the oils. Hippocrates, Pliny, Jesus, Socrates—all were proponents of essential oil usage, and some of the methods that they utilized are forever written in ancient texts.

In the Far East, processes of using aromatics flourished. The Chinese developed trade routes to India and other countries of the world to trade, buy, and sell oils, herbs, and spices. Japan further increased the use of essential oils through their distillation processes.

The English, the Italians, and the Spanish soon got in on the lucrative spice and oil trades. More knowledge of essential oil healing properties spread to almost every country in the world. These nations brought their knowledge of essential oils to the Americas, where it flourishes today.

Essential oils were used as currency in many areas of the world and were thought to be worth more than gold. Expeditions to discover new lands were developed due to the oil and spice trades. Because of these ambitious and adventurous people, the various cultures and countries of the world worked together to reach new and distant lands to obtain the precious oils.

Millions of lives have been saved throughout history by ancient doctors, shamans, and healers discovering therapeutic properties in plants, and then condensing those plants into oils that work to eradicate certain diseases, treat mental illnesses, heal infections, and reduce pain. I believe we can learn so much from our ancestors about healing inside and out by using essential oils.

Essential oils have been used in every religion on earth at one time or another. History shows us that herbs, oils, and plants have been closely tied to numerous worship rituals and rites. Many of those religions continue to use essential oils today to have a closer connection with their higher power, increase emotional responses of faith, and develop their own soul's journey.

How to Use This Book

People today want to heal from the inside out without relying on pharmaceuticals or chemicals that can often have devastating side effects. They want natural ways to incorporate emotional, mental, and spiritual healing into their lives and the lives of their friends and families. People the world over are turning to more natural, healthy, and simple ways of healing. *Essential Oils for Emotional Well-Being* shows how uncomplicated it can be to add natural healing to your lifestyle. The design and layout of this book is a simple and easy format that can be used by anyone.

This book is divided into chapters to give the reader easy accessibility in various categories based on conditions, emotions, needs, desires, or devotion, providing ease in locating what you need or desire. Each condition, emotion, need, desire, or devotion is followed by recipes that can be used to help with that condition. The recipes vary widely in each section to give you the options to use what essential oils you may have on hand.

A list of essential oils is provided after each condition. This list of oils is alphabetized and contains the most common essential oils used for that particular condition. Oftentimes, an oil from this list can be substituted in the recipes to replace an oil that you may not have available. Each of the oils contain therapeutic properties that work well for that particular condition.

At the end of this book, you will find appendices to help with the comprehension of technical terms, therapeutic properties, warnings, and other information regarding use. Becoming more familiar with these terms can help you to understand the recipes and explanations given throughout the book.

CHAPTER I
Essential Oils and the Emotions: Basic Use

$\mathcal{E}$ssential oils and the emotions have a huge impact on one another. This book will explain to you how the oils work on the emotions and how they can counteract or increase certain emotional responses in our systems—from "anger to worship." Using essential oils for emotional and spiritual needs dates back thousands of years.

Essential oils are created from plants, trees, herbs, fruit, and flowers. They are distilled, usually by steam distillation. The process involves placing the flowers or other plant material over steam. The steam releases all of the moisture and oils from the plant that then rise into the air. This moisture is captured and cooled. Since oil and water don't mix, the oil is separated from the water as it settles and cools. The oil is bottled and sold as essential oils. This is a simple explanation, but the process is quite involved and detailed. This is the most common process for making essential oils. There are actually several ways to remove the oils from the plants such as cold distillation, alcohol absorption (effleurage), and expression.

Essential oils are made up of molecules that contain various therapeutic properties. These properties have been studied, researched, and cataloged by scientists so that we can understand which healing actions are produced by which essential oils. I have listed the prominent therapeutic properties that work with each essential oil in the appendix section of this book.

These molecular wonders enter our body through the limbic system by the aromas and through our skin when we apply them. Hair follicles, sweat glands, and pores are very receptive to transmitting the oils from our skin directly into the bloodstream and into our very cells. At this point they are transmitted to the sites of need, much like aspirin or medicine is transported through the body.

When essential oils reach our brain, certain parts such as the hypothalamus, glands, neurotransmitters, and hormones are affected by the introduction of the cells containing the therapeutic properties. Our memories are sparked, our emotions are changed, and our brain reacts accordingly.

Therefore, when you are feeling stressed, sad, hyper, or any number of emotions, you can counteract those emotions with essential oils. Diffuse them, rub them on, or add them to the bathwater. It only takes a few drops to stimulate your limbic system and provide you with the needed responses. Even just opening the bottle and inhaling the wonderful aromas can have quick responses by our brains.

The main problem these days is trying to decide which brand to purchase, not how to find them. The age-old adage of "you get what you pay for" applies largely to the quality of essential oils. If you see a huge 16-fluid-ounce bottle of frankincense oil for $4 and a ½-fluid-ounce bottle for $34, you can pretty much guess which one is the real deal. Essential oils are usually derived from plants from the countries that the plants grow in naturally. Sometimes this can be extremely expensive, but well worth the price, as the oils in the plant grown in the native country will have better oils, more oils, and more therapeutic properties than if you grow them in your own backyard.

If you are purchasing oils for the aroma or to run in your diffuser, then a cheap oil will work well for you. If you are purchasing an oil for healing, then you would want to pay a little more to ensure you get a better oil. I buy all brands of oils and have them separated into various groups: cheap ones to run for aromas, medium-priced oils for everyday needs, and expensive oils for healing. I never turn down an essential oil. I can use them all for one thing or another.

But First: Tips and Warnings

Essential oils are fun. If you heed warnings and experiment cautiously, then you will be on your way to health, healing, and happiness with your aromatherapy. Before we dive into the main section of the book focused on oils for specific circumstances, we will first explore some of the basics. The unique warnings that may be present for individual oils can be viewed in the references section at the end of the book. There you will also find a glossary of definitions for technical terms that will come up throughout the book.

- I am not a licensed physician or a diagnostician and have had no medical training. I cannot condone using essential oils with any medications or illnesses without your doctor's or medical team's consent. Many medications and essential oils counteract each other or can cause serious consequences if used together. Consult with your doctor before beginning any essential oil regimen if you are on any medications or have been diagnosed with any diseases.

- Essential oils come in various strengths, potencies, and price ranges. Check with your friends, read reviews, and find outside sources to help you determine which brand is best for you. I like to use cheap essential oils in my diffuser, medium-grade and average-priced essential oils for my moods and minor ailments, and expensive clinical-grade essential oils for any more serious medical needs.

- Before you take any essential oils internally, ensure that the brand you are swallowing was made for ingesting. Some essential oils can burn a hole in your esophagus and stomach and even lead to fatal consequences. Please do your research before ever taking an essential oil by mouth. Some manufacturers state that their oils are safe for internal consumption, but most do not. If you decide to ingest essential oils, you should be under the guidance of a certified aromatherapist.

- Lock your essential oils up and away from children. Some essential oils can poison, burn, or scar a child, or cause devastating consequences and even death. Always ensure when giving some essential oils that you have the manufacturer's assurance that the oil will not harm the child. Never, ever, leave essential oils out and unattended or where a child can get to them. Never use essential oils on infants or toddlers without professional guidance.

• Essential oils should always be handled with care. Never apply to mucus membranes, sensitive areas such as eyes, genitals, or inner ears, and never apply directly to an open wound. Use caution at all times when using essential oils.

• Store your essential oils in a cool, dark area, such as a medicine cabinet or a cabinet that you can lock if there are children in the home. I like to use dark amber or green bottles to store my oils in. Sunlight can destroy the therapeutic properties in essential oils. Most oils will last for years if stored properly.

• Always use a carrier oil, milk, or some other recommended substance when diluting essential oils. Carrier oils can include (but are not limited to) sesame oil, grape seed oil, olive oil, avocado oil, jojoba oil, apricot seed oil, coconut oil, or any oil good for the skin and body. Some essential oils can be used neat (without carrier oil), but these are few. Always use extreme caution when handling essential oils.

• A patch test is the best way to determine if you are allergic to essential oils. Combine a mixture of 3–4 drops of essential oil with one teaspoon of carrier oil. Apply a small amount to an area of your skin. Do not bathe or get the area wet during the 12-hour waiting period. At the end of 12 hours look at the spot; if it is red, swollen, itchy, or looks unlike the rest of your surrounding skin, then you can assume you are allergic, or at least have a sensitivity to that particular oil and should not use it at all. If you have allergies to certain plants, you can be assured that you are also allergic to the essential oil from that same plant.

• If you are pregnant, nursing, think you might be pregnant, experience high blood pressure or low blood pressure, suffer from kidney issues, epilepsy, seizures, asthma, liver issues, heart problems, or any other illness or condition, you should check with a physician before taking any essential oils, to ensure that they won't affect your medications or your condition. Before taking an essential oil, read appendix 1 and do some online research to ensure your particular condition will not be affected.

• Essential oils contain therapeutic properties that can be damaged by heat. Use a diffuser that does not use heat to make steam, but uses a type of sound wave or vibration method. Ensure other oils, or water that your essential oils are added to, have been allowed to cool slightly to preserve the integrity of your oils.

- Children are especially vulnerable to the effects of essential oils. Ensure that milk is always added to their bath time rituals with essential oils. Milk will disperse the oils throughout the bath water and helps to prevent the oils from adhering to the skin and possibly causing a burn. Never use essential oils on a child under the age of four years, unless specified to do so by your physician.

- Never give essential oils to pets, as some oils that are safe for humans are toxic to pets. Ensure through your veterinarian that the oils you wish to use on your pets are safe for them. Never leave oils unattended where pets can reach them.

Where to Purchase

Essential oils can be purchased from a wide variety of places. When I first started using essential oils, they were very hard to locate, and once you found a place that sold essential oils, it became a frantic effort to purchase every one of them before the business was gone. Today, essential oils are sold online, in retail outlets, health food stores, and even huge chain department stores.

It is easier than ever to research the companies that sell the oils. Do they practice organic farming? Do they work entirely with essential oils or do they mass produce a variety of products? You can find all the information about a company online and determine if this is the right place for you to purchase your oils. Many countries around the world use false advertising to sell their oils. Ensure that the company you choose is ethical.

Many more essential oil companies are selling their products through home-based services. There are essential oil parties, essential oil product catalogs, and every town in America has people who sell essential oils through home-based marketing. Check them all out. You may find your newest favorite brand.

Labels

Learn to read labels on any oil that you purchase. Just because the label says "100 percent pure" does not necessarily mean 100 percent pure essential oil. It could mean 100 percent rose oil AND olive oil. Read the ingredients as well. There should only be one ingredient, and that would be the essential oil.

Occasionally, you will want to buy an essential oil that has been diluted with another oil. In these instances, the pure essential oil may be too expensive to purchase as a 100 percent straight oil, such as rose oil. Rose oil can cost upwards of $800 for a fraction of an ounce. So, buying this oil in a blend would be the best economically; otherwise, most of us could not ever afford to own a bottle of rose oil or some of the other pricier oils.

Buying blends that are already diluted with a carrier oil and ready to use right out of the bottle is very popular today. Many essential oil companies use their own recipes and add the carrier oil to the bottle for you. Just be sure when you are buying a blended or a straight essential oil that you differentiate between the two. Most blends can be applied directly to the skin from the bottle, but straight essential oils must be diluted before being applied.

The labels should direct you on how to use the oil, how often, and if it is 100 percent oil or if it has been mixed with a blend. Ensure that you are not using "fragrance oil" in your recipes instead of essential oils. Fragrance oils use chemicals to develop the aromas of the oils, and they do not contain therapeutic properties.

You can learn a lot about an oil from reading the label. Essential oils are fun and easy to use, as long as you are aware of what you are using and heed all of the tips and warnings associated with that particular oil.

Brands

There are hundreds of brands of essential oils. The government does not regulate labeling of essential oils that are to be used topically. Any company can put the words "100 percent essential oils" on their label, especially if they don't have strict advertising policies in their countries. You do want to make sure that you are buying 100 percent pure essential oils, so the best way to do this is to check the ingredients. It should only have one ingredient, and that would be the oil. If it has another word on there, then it is not 100 percent essential oil.

In the essential oil world market, you do actually get what you pay for. If you find a giant bottle of lavender essential oil, for example, and it is $5, then you are pretty much assured that you are not getting true essential oil. Many companies cut their essential oils with another, cheaper oil or use chemically derived fragrance oil. In these cheaper oils, you will not get the therapeutic properties that you are looking for.

Choosing a particular brand of essential oil is a personal preference. I personally use all of them. I use the cheap, off-the-shelf essential oils for my diffuser every day or for mixing up blends just for the aroma. I use the medium-grade essential oils for monitoring my moods or for simple everyday ailments. My very good essential oils I use for more serious situations. I never turn down an oil. I find a usage for all of them.

I often research companies that sell essential oils. I look for the plants to be indigenous to the areas of the world where they commonly grow. I like to buy oils that are organic and wholesome. Of course, I want clinical grade oils that can be used for healing. Some of my favorite brands of essential oils include Ovvio Oils, SunRose Aromatics, and Florihana. They meet all of my requirements for top-of-the-line essential oils and they are of true clinical grade and are ethically produced.

Try various brands of essential oils for your needs. Make notes about how the brands worked for you. You will soon find yourself turning more and more to a particular brand, or to multiple brands. There are some great oils on the market today, but there are some bad ones as well. What works well for one person may not work for another. Use your own judgment and get to know the companies that sell the oils.

Storage

Essential oils should be stored away from direct sunlight and heat. Sunlight will decrease the preserving actions in the oils. Using dark-colored bottles to store your oils and blends in is considered to be the optimal storage solution. Certain products, such as vitamin E oil and benzoin, can preserve your recipes and blends. That is why these are included in so many of the recipes in this book. Refrigerate your blends when requested in the recipes, otherwise they can have a great shelf life if stored in a cool/ dark area. I have a shelf in one of my closets that is devoted entirely to the storage of essential oils. I can shut the door, and my oils reside in total darkness. I also like to pick up medicine cabinets at flea markets, and I store my ready-made blends in them. Then they are easy to locate when I need them, and I can control the light that gets to them.

If an essential oil is stored properly and is a good brand, some of them can last many years. Take care of your oils, and ensure that they are out of reach of pets and children. Essential oils should never be left out on a counter or where pets and children can reach them. You and your essential oils can last many years together with proper storage.

Carrier Oils and Their Uses

A carrier oil is the oil we use to dilute the essential oils before applying them to our bodies. Essential oils are often too strong for the direct application to the skin. The oils must be diluted by mixing with an agent that will be readily absorbable by the skin, and the oils listed below are perfect for combining with essential oils. The carrier oil must be good for the skin, absorbable, and not have an overpowering aroma.

Essential oils can be applied to just about any area of the body, once they are diluted with a carrier oil. Studies were carried out by placing an essential oil mixed with a carrier oil onto the soles of the feet. Within a few minutes, the essential oil was detected in every cell in the body. Never apply essential oils on mucus membranes, open wounds, eyeballs, genitals, inside ears, or other sensitive areas.

Below, I am listing my favorite carrier oils. Experiment with your carrier oils and see which ones you like best! My general rule of thumb is to use ½ teaspoon carrier oil per 5–8 drops essential oil. Mix it, rub it on, and you're good to go!

Essential oils can burn as the properties are very strong, and must be cut with another substance. I have given a particular type of carrier oil in some of the recipes, but in most of them I leave it up to you to decide which carrier oil works best for you and your situation.

Take the same precautions with carrier oils that you would with essential oils. Read the labels to determine if it is 100 percent pure oil, or if it has been cut with a cheaper oil. Note the expiration dates, the ingredients, and use your eyes to determine if the oil looks clear or cloudy. Always smell your carrier oil before adding an essential oil to it. Carrier oils give a bitter aroma once they have turned rancid. Ensure your carrier oil is fresh and pure before mixing with your precious essential oils.

Sweet Almond Oil

I like sweet almond oil because it is cheap, readily available, and I use a lot of it! It's loaded with vitamins, so it's good for your skin. Almond oil will last a year on the shelf. It has lots of protein and is great to use in massage oils.

Apricot Kernel Oil

This oil is great for dry, aged skin (like mine). It works wonders as a moisturizing lotion and is used in antiaging products worldwide. It's loaded with vitamin A and is a good base for healing products.

Grape Seed Oil

One of my favorite carrier oils. Very inexpensive. It doesn't have as great of a shelf life as most of the other oils, but I use it up within 6 months of buying it, so that's OK. It has vitamins A and E, so it's perfect for your skin. The molecules are very tiny and are absorbed by the skin rapidly.

Jojoba Oil

This oil is amazing for all skin types, and it's especially good for skin conditions. It will keep forever on the shelf and mixes beautifully with essential oils and other carrier oils. It's great for the hair, scalp, and skin. I am crazy for jojoba oil, even though it is a little pricey. I use this oil for more serious ailments or skin issues.

Olive Oil

I really don't like using olive oil, as it is thick and greasy, but I have been known to use it in a pinch. It will last 1–2 years on the shelf, so it has a pretty good shelf life. It does have an odor that will come through when mixed with essential oils, but it will work to transmit your essential oils into your body and brain! Read the ingredient label thoroughly, as olive oil is often cut with cheaper oils. The label will indicate if it is 100 percent pure olive oil.

Sesame Oil

This oil works well for lowering the vata dosha (which I am most in abundance of, therefore, I use it almost every day). It has protein, vitamins, and minerals, so it is very good for the body and the skin. Sesame is also what I use for oil pulling, which is gargling and swishing the oil through the mouth. The oil is a magnet for toxins, which adhere to the oil. Spit the oil out after swishing. Sesame oil has a pretty long shelf life; it never has gone rancid on me, even after a year or two.

Methods of Using Recipes

The numerous recipes in this book are easy to make and use and they usually contain items that can be found throughout your home. The basic recipes are formulas that I have worked with for many years and found to be the most effective at dispersing oils to the home or body. The following is a brief description of the various methods of the recipes used throughout this book. These methods correspond to the recipe list at the beginning of the book.

Bath

This is one of the most enjoyable ways to use your essential oils. The oils can enter through your skin and nasal passages and provide you with a beautiful healing experience. Never fill the tub with extremely hot water, as the heat can destroy any therapeutic properties in the oils. A lukewarm bath is the best method to use to maintain the integrity of the oils. The oils will float on top of the water, adhering to the skin; to help disperse the oils, it is common to add a tablespoon of milk to the bathwater. This step will allow the oils to mix with the water.

Bath Bombs

Bath and shower bombs are fun and easy to make. They are made from ingredients that harden after the essential oils are added. Once you settle into the tub, they can be placed in with you, and they give off a fizzing action that releases the essential oils into the water and air. Shower bombs can be placed onto the floor of the shower where the water will cause them to fizz and release their aromas into the air. Bath and shower bombs make great gifts and can be molded into a variety of shapes and sizes.

Bath Salts

Bath salts are a fun way to get healing salts into your bath. They are inexpensive to make, beautiful as gifts, and give a spa-like atmosphere to the bath ritual. Depending on the type of salts you use, you can get different healing benefits from the salts. Epsom and pink Himalayan salts provide great muscle pain relief due to the minerals inherent in these salts. Discover what salts bring the effect you desire. Ensure that the water is not so hot as to destroy the beneficial effects of the properties in the oils.

Compress

A compress is an age-old healing method whereby the oils are mixed with either a carrier oil or water and applied to a large square of gauze or linen. The compress can be left on until it is no longer comfortable or applied as directed.

Diffuser

A diffuser imparts healing and delightful aromas throughout the home, office, or wherever you plug one in. Ensure that your diffuser does not use heat to make steam. Cold diffusers are the only type of diffuser that won't hurt the oils. Only cold water should be added to a diffuser, unless otherwise specified by the manufacturer. Cleaning your diffuser according to manufacturer's directions can add years to your diffuser. Each diffuser holds a different amount of water and essential oils. Ensure you are using the specified amounts. There are various methods for turning the water and oils into a fine mist that drifts in the air and benefits those who come into contact.

Footbath

A footbath requires a large receptacle, such as a large bowl or pan. Using a footbath can deliver essential oils throughout the body, muscles, tendons, and areas specified in the directions. The feet are considered to be one of the best vehicles to distribute essential oils to the rest of the body. The water should be lukewarm and comfortable. Ensure you have a towel handy to dry your feet on when you take them out of the footbath so you don't slip and fall. A teaspoon of milk added to the water will help disperse the oils throughout the water, ensuring they won't adhere to your skin. The recipes indicate which oils, and how much of each, should be used for each various condition.

Hand Rub

The hand rub is one of the most common ways to use essential oils; it is easy and effective. Combining a carrier oil and essential oils, briskly rub the oils into the hands. Use a small amount during the day, as it can be absorbed readily into the skin. At night, before bed, use a thicker application of the oils to the hands and cover with gloves. This way the oils can penetrate the skin all during the night while you are sleeping.

Inhale

Inhaling essential oil aromas can vastly affect the moods and emotions by changing the molecules in our brains and in the limbic system. There are devices that you can purchase, such as nasal inhalers, that are effective and affordable. Other than a nasal inhaler, placing a drop of the oils onto a tissue or into the palm of your hand can be just as effective as any apparatus. Simply close a nostril and breathe in the aroma with the open nostril. The effects are quick, and it only takes 1 drop of oil.

Laundry Detergent

Mix the ingredients together in a small bowl or container. Stir well. I like to add about 16 drops to a ½ gallon container of liquid laundry detergent. It is not recommended to add essential oils to powdered laundry detergent until each usage. Add the manufacturer's recommended amount of oil-infused laundry detergent to each load in the washer. Store remainder in a glass jar with a tight-fitting lid in a cool, dark area for up to 1 year.

Linen Powder

Making linen powder is easy and fun. Various essential oils are applied to the powder to enhance the needed benefits. Using a mason jar with holes poked into the lid is the most common method. The powder is sprinkled under the bed sheets or into the pillowcases to impart the sleep-inducing and calming effects of the oils throughout the night. You can use a small piece of plastic wrap between the lid and the band to cover the holes in your mason jar when not in use.

Lip Balm

Add the vitamin E, the essential oils, beeswax, and other ingredients, and stir quickly. With a spoon, drip a drop of the mixture onto the counter and let set for 1 minute. Pull your finger through the drop and check for consistency. If mixture is too thin, add more beeswax; if it is too thick, add more oil. Once desired consistency is acquired, immediately pour into small balm container (glass or metal) with a lid. After mixture cools, cover and store in a cool, dark area for up to 6 months.

Lotion

Add the recommended amount of essential oils to any brand of mild unscented lotion. Whisk until thoroughly mixed. Apply lotion to body as needed. Store unused portion in a jar with a tight-fitting lid in a cool, dark area for up to 1 month.

Massage Oil

Purchasing a massage oil can be quite expensive. Making your own is easy, cost efficient, and can provide you with many healing benefits. In a bowl, just add the essential oils to the carrier oil specified and whisk. Pour into a bottle, label, and date. Warming the oil by rubbing it briskly between the hands before applying will make the recipient feel more comfortable as it is being applied to the skin.

Neat

"Neat" is the term given to an essential oil application whereby the oil is applied directly to the skin, without cutting it with a carrier oil first. Only a few essential oils are recommended to be applied in this manner. Most oils will burn or irritate the skin if not diluted. Ensure through your doctor or a certified aromatherapist which essential oils can be applied neat for your condition.

Ointment

An ointment is a mixture of ingredients, usually containing a small amount of beeswax, that is heated, cooled, and applied to the skin. After heating the carrier oil, beeswax, and the other ingredients, it is best to add the essential oils after the heated oil has cooled slightly. Once all the ingredients are whisked together, it should be poured into smaller containers quickly, as it will thicken into a gel-like consistency. Ointment can be applied with or without a bandage or covering, depending on the site area and how it comes into contact with clothing and furniture.

Roller Bottle

Essential oils can be mixed with carrier oils, or other ingredients, and poured into roller bottles for easy access, usage, and storage. Roller bottles are convenient to carry in a purse, car, or to leave in a medicine cabinet or office desk. It's important to always label your bottles so that you can tell which bottle works for what need.

Rub

Pour the essential oils, carrier oil, and any remaining ingredients into a small glass container, bowl, or jar. Swirl or whisk to mix the ingredients, and apply lightly to the area desired, such as pressure points, neck, soles of feet, temples, or chest. Protect furniture and clothing from stains by wearing an old T-shirt. Keep the essential oil mixture away from open wounds, mucus membranes, genitals, eyes, and sensitive areas. Repeat application as needed, usually 2–3 times daily. Store unused portion in a glass jar or container with a tight-fitting lid in a cool, dark area for up to 6 months.

Salve

A salve is a very thick ointment that stays in place on the skin when applied. Beeswax is the optimal way to thicken the ingredients. The carrier oil and beeswax are heated until the wax is melted. After cooling slightly, the essential oils are added, and the mixture is poured into containers with lids. When applying to the skin, a bandage or linen is usually used to cover the area, as the salve can sometimes damage clothing or furniture. Salves have a long shelf life if vitamin E oil is added as a preservative.

Smelling Salts

Smelling salts bring back ancient days when ladies would carry a vial of smelling salts in their "reticules" and take a whiff when they felt they were going to faint. In actuality, smelling salts are a great way to quickly get the essential oils to pass the blood/ brain barrier and get those healing molecules straight into our systems. The salts preserve the oils and keep those healing properties active for a long period of time.

Spray

Sprays are an easy and effective way to impart the aromas into the air or onto the body. The important thing to remember about sprays is that they must be shaken vigorously before each usage, as the oils and water will definitely separate when sitting. Sprays are one of the most common ways to use essential oils because of the readily available ingredients, water and oils.

Spritzer

A spritzer is made with fewer oils than a spray, thereby lending themselves as the perfect vehicle for spraying the body or hair. Spritzers must be shaken well before using, as the oils and water will separate during sitting.

Sugar Scrub

Combine ingredients without mashing too much. Spread paste onto skin or area desired and rub in lightly. Do not apply to genitals, eyes, sensitive areas, or mucus membranes. Sugar scrub should never be applied to the face. Let set for 1 minute, and then gently rinse off. Keep in a mason jar with a tight-fitting lid in a cool, dark area for up to 1 month.

Wrap

Mix ingredients together into a small bowl or container. Apply the mixture onto a long, rectangle piece of muslin, linen, gauze, or cotton. Wrap the treated material around the wrist, knee, ankle, etc. Leave wrap on for at least 15 minutes. Store remainder of ingredients in a jar with a tight-fitting lid for up to 30 days.

CHAPTER 2
Chakras and Doshas

Some of the various emotional and spiritual needs in this book may have terms that you are not familiar with, such as the "chakras" and the "doshas." These ancient energies are defined and discussed in this book and help us to figure out what areas of our minds, spirits, and souls we need to work on, and how to reach the point where we can finally know that we are on the right track to good spiritual, physical, and mental health. Learning about your chakras and doshas is fun and easy. Treating and balancing the chakras and doshas is a lifetime quest.

We all have chakras and doshas, which are the characteristics of our personality, mentality, energy centers, and physical makeup. The chakras and doshas are important for us to understand in order to have optimal physical and mental health. In this book we will take a journey through the history, explanations, and differences in the chakras and doshas that make up our energy and our dispositions. Recipes are included in this chapter to assist you with balancing and opening your chakras and doshas and to help you achieve the results you desire in your life.

Introduction to Chakras

Our chakras are the seven energy sources in our bodies that are believed to connect our spiritual, mental, and physical selves. Knowledge of the chakras has existed for over three thousand years in various cultures. People have believed throughout time that if your chakras are out of balance, it can have a negative impact on various areas of your life. Many people are stuck in a particular rut in their lives due to issues with one of their chakras. Conversely, emotional and traumatic events in our lives can affect our chakras. Learning about the chakras and working on balancing them out can help in numerous areas of your body and bring overall balance, peace of mind, a closer connection to Spirit, satisfaction in your soul, connections with loved ones, and harmony to your life.

The chakras were first discovered and used as a guide for optimal health in India over three thousand years ago. Since that time, the use of balancing chakras as a health tool has been used in cultures worldwide. Ancient sacred Hindu texts, the Upanishads, are the oldest texts we have today that discuss chakras and the energies of the human body.

The chakras are invisible energy centers that control our thoughts, actions, moods, anxieties, desires, physical bodies, needs, and everything about ourselves. These "subtle energies" are in seven areas of our body, all along the spinal canal. The chakras lay at the base of the spine, at our sacrum, at our navel, at our heart, at our throat, at our forehead, and at the top or crown of our heads. Learning which chakra does what and how to work on individual chakras is beneficial to our mental and physical health.

Each of the seven chakras has a meaning. For example, the root chakra, *Muladhara*, is responsible for grounding us. We may be stuck in this chakra because our vata is too high, we don't meditate, or we did not have a good family base as an infant, among other reasons. There are a number of grounding activities, herbs, essential oils, and diets we can use in order to have more grounding in our lives, thereby balancing our root chakra. If we are stuck in our base chakra, we might be unable to have strong attachments, be frivolous with money, be unable to sit still, have ADD, or be generally too hyperactive. Working on different ways to give us grounding can open up and heal the root chakra and take care of many issues in our lives.

So much mental and physical healing and clarity can come from working our way up through the chakras, opening each of them up, and exploring the various aspects such as communication, heart, sexual proclivity, and other aspects of the chakras. Look at the chakras and decide where you are stuck and which one you need to work on to give yourself the best possible outcome in your life.

The seven chakras are:

- *Muladhara*, the root chakra
- *Svadhistana*, the sacral chakra
- *Manipura*, the solar plexus chakra
- *Anahata*, the heart chakra
- *Visuddha*, the throat chakra
- *Ajna*, the third eye chakra
- *Sahasrara*, the crown chakra

Learning about the chakras' influences on our lives, personalities, and health can be so beneficial to us. It can help us to lead fuller, longer lives. Say, for example, you have trouble communicating on all levels, with your career, with your spouse, and with your friends. Maybe you have issues with telling people how you really feel. Then you are probably blocked in your throat chakra. Learning what essential oils you can use to help unblock your throat chakra can help you find and correct your issues with communication.

Understanding the chakras and how they relate to our lives takes a lifetime of study, work, and research. You can have a basic grasp through this book on how you can use essential oils for certain emotions to help unblock certain chakras. Hopefully, this will spur a desire in you to learn all you can about chakras and work throughout your life to bring your chakras into balance.

Below are seven sections, one for each chakra. An overall view of each of the chakras, the Sanskrit word for that chakra, and a definition of that particular chakra is given to help you familiarize yourself with your chakras. Areas of your life that can be affected by the blockage of a chakra are listed, followed by the essential oils that are used to open and heal this chakra. Several recipes are in each category that can work to open the chakras and bring particular results into your life.

Root Chakra (Muladhara)

Located at the tailbone, the root chakra is our first chakra. It is what grounds us. It is responsible for us feeling safe and secure. The essential oils in this recipe are noted to have benefits in making us feel grounded and securing our root chakra so that we feel connected to the world. Balancing our root chakra helps to rid us of those flighty, anxiety-producing, and impulsive feelings. Oftentimes abandonment issues stem from our root chakra. Grounding ourselves can help us to feel much less anxious and fearful and to appreciate the simple things in life. The root chakra is associated with our basic human needs: food, clothing, and shelter. Hardcore addictions are associated with the root chakra.

Essential Oils

Benzoin, clematis, frankincense, myrrh, patchouli, rosemary, sandalwood, and ylang-ylang

Root Linen Powder

Bring your root chakra into balance while you sleep. This powder will help you to relax, and you can drift off to sleep knowing that you are firmly rooted to the earth. The therapeutic properties in this blend include sedative, analgesic, antidepressant, and tranquilizing agents.

Yield: ¼ cup

RECIPE

7 drops ylang-ylang oil

5 drops frankincense oil

3 drops clematis oil

4 drops vitamin E oil

¼ cup cornstarch

Place the ingredients into a mason jar, stirring well with a whisk. Carefully poke holes into the lid, use this as a shaker, and shake the ingredients into pillowcases or under sheet areas as needed. You can get a piece of plastic wrap and place it over the jar and

under the lid to keep powder from spilling out when not in use. Store in a glass jar or container with a tight-fitting lid in a cool, dark, and dry area for up to 3 months.

Grounding Air Diffuser Blend

The essential oils in this blend are reported to help a person feel more grounded and safe with their calming, sedative, and harmonizing properties. Run this in your diffuser while you are at home all day or at work, and let go of that flighty, anxious, nervous feeling.

Yield: 1 application

RECIPE
2 drops sandalwood oil
2 drops frankincense oil
2 drops ylang-ylang oil
Water

Follow your directions for using essential oils in your particular brand of diffuser. Ensure that your diffuser does not use heat but runs by vibration, sound waves, or another cold-steam type of process. Choose the essential oils needed for your condition, then add water and oils to the diffuser. Run your diffuser as needed to permeate the air with therapeutic properties and achieve the results you desire.

Grounding Spray

When you are feeling like you don't know where to turn and you can't make a simple decision, use this spray to ground you and bring your life into balance. These essential oils are known for their grounding due to the natural components such as nervine, sedative, aphrodisiac, and antidepressant therapeutic properties.

Yield: 2 fluid ounces

RECIPE
3 drops rosemary oil
4 drops patchouli oil
3 drops myrrh oil

3 drops vitamin E oil

1 tablespoon witch hazel

2 fluid ounces water

Add all ingredients to a dark-colored spray bottle. Check for material steadfastness before spraying on fabric. Shake the bottle and spray onto area desired, such as body, hair, home, car, or office. Do not spray into or on open wounds, genitals, eyes, or mucus membranes. Store in a cool, dark area for up to 3 months. Shake well before each use to combine the ingredients.

Grounding Bath

Soak in these essential oils and, when you come out of the bath, they will help you to feel that you do have the ability to concentrate, focus, and feel grounded. These essential oils can assist you in being thankful that you are alive and have a home, food, and clothing. These are the basics of grounding oneself. The components at work in this recipe include sedative, calming, tranquilizing, and antidepressant properties.

Yield: 1 application

Recipe

6 drops frankincense oil

6 drops sandalwood oil

3 drops ylang-ylang oil

1 tablespoon carrier oil

1 tablespoon milk (optional for adults, recommended for children)

As you begin to fill the tub with water, pour the chosen essential oils and carrier oil into the running water. Run a warm, not hot, bath. Water that is too hot will cause the essential oils to dissipate. You may add 1 tablespoon of milk to the water; this ensures that the essential oils will not stick to your skin, but will mix with the water. You may soak in the water as long as you are comfortable. Dry your feet well once you get out of the water, as the oils will cause them to be slippery, increasing your chances of falling. Rinse the tub of any remaining oils.

Root Bath Salts

Sometimes we view bath salts as an indulgence, but when you couple them with these grounding essential oils, you will emerge a new and more focused person. Therapeutic properties such as antidepressant, antirheumatic, sedative, and anti-inflammatory abilities work together to bring a sense of calmness and rootedness to our very cores.

Yield: 3 cups

RECIPE
8 drops frankincense oil

5 drops myrrh oil

5 drops clematis oil

2 tablespoons carrier oil

5 drops vitamin E oil

3 cups salts

1 tablespoon milk (optional for adults, recommended for children)

Use any type of salt you prefer: pink Himalayan salt, sea salt, Epsom salts, etc. In a small container, add the essential oils to the desired type of salt. Stir until well blended. Screw lid onto container tightly. Leave mixture in a dark area for 24 hours and then stir mixture again. Run the bathwater. Once the tub is full of water, you can add the milk, and then add ½ cup of the bath salt mixture to bathwater as you get into the tub. You may stay in the tub as long as the temperature is comfortable. Dry your feet well when you get out of the bath, as the oils are slippery and can cause you to fall. Store remainder in a glass jar or container with a tight-fitting lid in a cool, dark area for up to 3 months. These jars make attractive, inexpensive, and healing gifts!

Sacral Chakra (Svadhistana)

Located in our pelvic area, the sacral chakra is responsible for our creativity, sexual desire, and problem solving. It is our second chakra. These recipes and oils are reported to bring us to a closer relationship with our desires and creative aspects of our lives, and give us clear-headed insight into what event needs to take place to balance this particular chakra. The sacral chakra is also known as the pleasure chakra. Food addictions, shame, and guilt are associated with the sacral chakra.

Essential Oils

Bergamot, citrus oils, hibiscus, jasmine, lemon, mandarin, melissa, neroli, orange, and rose

Sacral Linen Powder

Sprinkle this powder under the sheets and bring balance to your love life. These essential oils are known for their aphrodisiacal and sedative properties.

Yield: 10–20 applications

RECIPE
6 drops neroli oil
6 drops hibiscus oil
6 drops rose oil
4 drops vitamin E oil
¼ cup cornstarch

Place the ingredients into a mason jar, stirring well with a whisk. Carefully poke holes into the lid, use this as a shaker, and shake the ingredients into pillowcases or under sheet areas as needed. You can get a piece of plastic wrap and place it over the jar and under the lid to keep powder from spilling out when not in use. Store in a glass jar or container with a tight-fitting lid in a cool, dark, and dry area for up to 3 months.

Sex in the Air

These essential oils will bring your body and mind together to help move your love life into a greater balance with your work and home life. The natural agents at work in this recipe are aphrodisiac, stimulant, antidepressant, and nervine properties.

Yield: 1 application

RECIPE
3 drops rose oil
3 drops jasmine oil

3 drops grapefruit oil

Water

Follow your directions for using essential oils in your particular brand of diffuser. Ensure that your diffuser does not use heat but runs by vibration, sound waves, or another cold-steam type of process. Choose the essential oils needed for your condition, then add water and oils to the diffuser. Run your diffuser as needed to permeate the air with therapeutic properties and achieve the results you desire.

Creativity Spray

If you need a boost in the creative department and want to think outside of the box, this spray will help you to focus on the creative areas of your life. Open your mind with this recipe and get going on that project. Some of the focusing components of this blend include tonic, antidepressant, and nervine properties.

Yield: 2 fluid ounces

RECIPE

4 drops neroli oil

3 drops melissa oil

3 drops sweet orange oil

3 drops vitamin E oil

1 tablespoon witch hazel

2 fluid ounces water

Add all ingredients to a dark-colored spray bottle. Check for material steadfastness before spraying on fabric. Shake the bottle and spray onto area desired, such as body, hair, home, car, or office. Do not spray into or on open wounds, genitals, eyes, or mucus membranes. Store in a cool, dark area for up to 3 months. Shake well before each use to combine the ingredients.

New Discoveries Bath

For the maximum benefits of these oils, two people should share this recipe together. Enjoy the creativity and imagination that is let loose by these essential oils and begin the journey for that sacral chakra healing that you crave. Boost your creative juices with these aphrodisiac, nervine, and tonic-inducing therapeutic properties.

Yield: 1 application

RECIPE
6 drops lemon oil
4 drops hibiscus oil
4 drops rose oil
1 tablespoon carrier oil
1 tablespoon milk (optional for adults, recommended for children)

As you begin to fill the tub with water, pour the chosen essential oils and carrier oil into the running water. Run a warm, not hot, bath. Water that is too hot will cause the essential oils to dissipate. You may add 1 tablespoon of milk to the water; this ensures that the essential oils will not stick to your skin, but will mix with the water. You may soak in the water as long as you are comfortable. Dry your feet well once you get out of the water, as the oils will cause them to be slippery, increasing your chances of falling. Rinse the tub of any remaining oils.

Sacral Bath Salts

Open a whole new world of creativity and desire by letting your imagination run loose with these essential oils. A little in your bath can go a long way in helping you learn to cope with your desires, open up about your needs, and increase your wilder, freer side. This blend contains aphrodisiac, tonic, stimulating, and aromatic therapeutic properties.

Yield: 3 cups

RECIPE
10 drops jasmine oil
5 drops neroli oil
5 drops rose oil
2 tablespoons carrier oil
3 cups salts

5 drops vitamin E oil

1 tablespoon milk (optional for adults, recommended for children)

Use any type of salt you prefer: pink Himalayan salt, sea salt, Epsom salts, etc. In a small container, add the essential oils to the desired type of salt. Stir until well blended. Screw lid onto container tightly. Leave mixture in a dark area for 24 hours and then stir mixture again. Run the bathwater. Once the tub is full of water, you can add the milk, and then add ½ cup of the bath salt mixture to bathwater as you get into the tub. You may stay in the tub as long as the temperature is comfortable. Dry your feet well when you get out of the bath, as the oils are slippery and can cause you to fall. Store remainder in a glass jar or container with a tight-fitting lid in a cool, dark area for up to 3 months. These jars make attractive, inexpensive, and healing gifts!

Solar Plexus Chakra (Manipura)

Located above the naval, the solar plexus chakra is our third chakra and is responsible for our arrogance and self-esteem. Many tendencies we have in our lives that lead us to have an imbalance in how we relate to the world around us originate with imbalances in the solar plexus chakra. These oils and recipes are made to help us increase our self-esteem, see others for how they truly are, and have more empathy toward those in need. This particular chakra is considered the one we should pay the most attention to and complete the most work on in order to balance all of our chakras and bring our lives to the point that we desire. Judgments, opinions, self-esteem, and confidence are associated with the solar plexus chakra.

Essential Oils

Chamomile, juniper, lemon, marjoram, peppermint, petitgrain, vetiver, and yarrow

Solar Plexus Linen Powder

Feel better about yourself when you wake up in the morning after basking all night in the aroma of the essential oils in this powder. You will be clearheaded, motivated and able to look others in the eye again. These essential oils will assist in helping you to possess more self-confidence and self-assuredness. This is the recipe to use when you have a big meeting or an interview coming up and you need to have that "I can do it" attitude. Full of nervine and sedative properties, this blend will help to lull you into a peaceful night's sleep so that you may awaken refreshed and empowered.

Yield: ¼ cup

RECIPE
5 drops petitgrain oil
6 drops chamomile oil
6 drops juniper oil
4 drops vitamin E oil
¼ cup cornstarch

Place the ingredients into a mason jar, stirring well with a whisk. Carefully poke holes into the lid, use this as a shaker, and shake the ingredients into pillowcases or under sheet areas as needed. You can get a piece of plastic wrap and place it over the jar and under the lid to keep powder from spilling out when not in use. Store in a glass jar or container with a tight-fitting lid in a cool, dark, and dry area for up to 3 months.

Confident Diffuser

Are you having a meeting today and need a boost of confidence? Run this diffuser at work and see how others react when you are feeling great and full of self-assuredness, and have the ability to put yourself and your ideas at the forefront of any conversation or meeting. The calming and soothing properties of this recipe will help to keep your thoughts focused and on task.

Yield: 1 application

RECIPE
3 drops yarrow oil
2 drops chamomile oil
2 drops lemon oil
Water

Follow your directions for using essential oils in your particular brand of diffuser. Ensure that your diffuser does not use heat but runs by vibration, sound waves, or another cold-steam type of process. Choose the essential oils needed for your condition, then add water and oils to the diffuser. Run your diffuser as needed to permeate the air with therapeutic properties and achieve the results you desire.

Self-Esteem Spray

Carry this spray with you everywhere you go and use the essential oils that are famous for boosting self-esteem. Regain that confidence and promote yourself by getting your solar plexus chakra back into balance. This recipe contains, anti-inflammatory, and antidepressant properties for a great, all-over feeling of well-being.

Yield: 2 fluid ounces

RECIPE

3 drops peppermint oil

3 drops petitgrain oil

2 drops vetiver oil

3 drops vitamin E oil

1 tablespoon witch hazel

2 fluid ounces water

Add all ingredients to a dark-colored spray bottle. Check for material steadfastness before spraying on fabric. Shake the bottle and spray onto area desired, such as body, hair, home, car, or office. Do not spray into or on open wounds, genitals, eyes, or mucus membranes. Store in a cool, dark area for up to 3 months. Shake well before each use to combine the ingredients.

I'm Worth Everything Bath

Time to get your solar plexus chakra into shape by using these essential oils. You are valuable and you are worth everything and it's time that you begin to feel that in your soul. Some of the agents at work in this blend include nervine, sedative, stomachic, calming, and tranquilizing components.

Yield: 1 application

RECIPE

6 drops juniper oil

3 drops marjoram oil

4 drops chamomile oil

1 tablespoon carrier oil

1 tablespoon milk (optional for adults, recommended for children)

As you begin to fill the tub with water, pour the chosen essential oils and carrier oil into the running water. Run a warm, not hot, bath. Water that is too hot will cause the essential oils to dissipate. You may add 1 tablespoon of milk to the water; this ensures that the essential oils will not stick to your skin, but will mix with the water. You may soak in the water as long as you are comfortable. Dry your feet well once you get out of the water, as the oils will cause them to be slippery, increasing your chances of falling. Rinse the tub of any remaining oils.

Solar Plexus Bath Salts

While taking this bath, give gratitude that you were made into such a wonderful person. These essential oils will have you feeling on top of the world and give you the confidence you need to accomplish anything and everything. Get the benefits you need from these natural properties including nervine, sedative, anti-inflammatory, and circulatory stimulating components.

Yield: 3 cups

RECIPE

8 drops yarrow oil

7 drops petitgrain oil

5 drops juniper oil

2 tablespoons carrier oil

5 drops vitamin E oil

3 cups salts

1 tablespoon milk (optional for adults, recommended for children)

Use any type of salt you prefer: pink Himalayan salt, sea salt, Epsom salts, etc. In a small container, add the essential oils to the desired type of salt. Stir until well blended. Screw lid onto container tightly. Leave mixture in a dark area for 24 hours and then stir mixture again. Run the bathwater. Once the tub is full of water, you can add the milk, and then add ½ cup of the bath salt mixture to bathwater as you get into the tub. You may stay in the tub as long as the temperature is comfortable. Dry your feet well when you get out of the bath, as the oils are slippery and can cause you to fall. Store remainder in a glass jar or container with a tight-fitting lid in a cool, dark area for up to 3 months. These jars make attractive, inexpensive, and healing gifts!

Heart Chakra (Anahata)

As expected, this chakra is the fourth and is located near the heart. The heart chakra not only assists us in giving and receiving love, but also allows us to heal from losing a loved one through abandonment, death, and separation. These oils and recipes are sure to assist us in dealing with past loves and securing our future loves through working on balancing the heart chakra. Courage, compassion, love of others, and self-love originate within the heart chakra.

Essential Oils
Bergamot, eucalyptus, holly, jasmine, melissa, pine, poppy, and rose

Find Love Linen Powder
Sleep on this essential oil blend and wake up feeling better about your future and not so focused on the past. Grieving is a natural process and should be explored in depth, but not to the detriment of our other loved ones or our livelihoods. Grieve, cry, pray, and do all you can to come out the other side a stronger person. Many components are inherent in this recipe to help you heal, including antidepressant, sedative, nervine, hypotensive, tonic, and aromatic therapeutic properties.

Yield: ¼ cup

RECIPE
7 drops melissa oil
5 drops bergamot oil
3 drops rose oil

4 drops vitamin E oil

¼ cup cornstarch

Place the ingredients into a mason jar, stirring well with a whisk. Carefully poke holes into the lid, use this as a shaker, and shake the ingredients into pillowcases or under sheet areas as needed. You can get a piece of plastic wrap and place it over the jar and under the lid to keep powder from spilling out when not in use. Store in a glass jar or container with a tight-fitting lid in a cool, dark, and dry area for up to 3 months.

Love is in the Air

After losing the love of your life, we are often plagued with thinking that we will never find love again; run this diffuser and focus on finding love again. These essential oils help us to realize our worth and give us hope for the future. These heart chakra balancing oils can heal and repair the imbalances you feel in your heart. A few of the therapeutic properties working to benefit you include aromatic, antidepressant, tonic, and nervine natural agents.

Yield: 1 application

RECIPE

3 drops poppy oil

2 drops rose oil

2 drops bergamot oil

Water

Follow your directions for using essential oils in your particular brand of diffuser. Ensure that your diffuser does not use heat but runs by vibration, sound waves, or another cold-steam type of process. Choose the essential oils needed for your condition, then add water and oils to the diffuser. Run your diffuser as needed to permeate the air with therapeutic properties and achieve the results you desire.

Conjuring Love Spray

Carry this spray with you and use it when you want to bring another person into tune with yourself. A one-sided love affair is not good for anyone, so get this little heart chakra blend together and use it often on yourself, and around the one you are attracted to. Balancing and healing your heart chakra is paramount to any future endeavors you wish to pursue. This blend opens the heart of all those who are encompassed by its aromas with aphrodisiac and tonic properties.

Yield: 2 fluid ounces

RECIPE
5 drops melissa oil
4 drops jasmine oil
3 drops rose oil
3 drops vitamin E oil
1 tablespoon witch hazel
2 fluid ounces water

Add all ingredients to a dark-colored spray bottle. Check for material steadfastness before spraying on fabric. Shake the bottle and spray onto area desired, such as body, hair, home, car, or office. Do not spray into or on open wounds, genitals, eyes, or mucus membranes. Store in a cool, dark area for up to 3 months. Shake well before each use to combine the ingredients.

Opening the Heart to Good Bath

These essential oils will help bring about feelings in the heart, and you will want to express and explore them. Immerse yourself in this little bit of luxury, try to concentrate on positive emotions that wash over you, and rid yourself of the negative feelings that can bar your heart from accepting love from others. Open yourself up to what is right in front of you while healing your heart chakra at the same time. Therapeutic properties in this recipe include aromatic and antidepressant agents.

Yield: 1 application

RECIPE
4 drops pine oil
4 drops holly oil
4 drops bergamot oil
1 tablespoon carrier oil
1 tablespoon milk (optional for adults, recommended for children)

As you begin to fill the tub with water, pour the chosen essential oils and carrier oil into the running water. Run a warm, not hot, bath. Water that is too hot will cause the essential oils to dissipate. You may add 1 tablespoon of milk to the water; this ensures that the essential oils will not stick to your skin, but will mix with the water. You may soak in the water as long as you are comfortable. Dry your feet well once you get out of the water, as the oils will cause them to be slippery, increasing your chances of falling. Rinse the tub of any remaining oils.

Open My Heart Bath Salts

These bath salts have essential oils that will help to open your heart to accepting the losses in your life and embracing new loves. Rid yourself of those feelings of grief that can be overwhelming and have you closing your heart to others. Be open, willing, and able to have connections with people, and eliminate that wall of steel you have built as protection.

Yield: 3 cups

RECIPE

9 drops bergamot oil

5 drops rose oil

5 drops holly oil

2 tablespoons carrier oil

5 drops vitamin E oil

3 cups salts

1 tablespoon milk (optional for adults, recommended for children)

Use any type of salt you prefer: pink Himalayan salt, sea salt, Epsom salts, etc. In a small container, add the essential oils to the desired type of salt. Stir until well blended. Screw lid onto container tightly. Leave mixture in a dark area for 24 hours and then stir mixture again. Run the bathwater. Once the tub is full of water, you can add the milk, and then add ½ cup of the bath salt mixture to bathwater as you get into the tub. You may stay in the tub as long as the temperature is comfortable. Dry your feet well when you get out of the bath, as the oils are slippery and can cause you

to fall. Store remainder in a glass jar or container with a tight-fitting lid in a cool, dark area for up to 3 months. These jars make attractive, inexpensive, and healing gifts!

Throat Chakra (Visuddha)

The fifth chakra is located at the throat. Balancing this chakra allows us to effectively communicate with those around us. The throat chakra is responsible for speaking, listening, writing, and all forms of communication. These oils and recipes are sure to assist us with opening lines of communication between our loved ones and us. Communication is the key to a successful relationship between you and humanity. Communication, feelings, desires, and repressed anger come from the throat chakra.

Essential Oils

Cosmos, geranium, German chamomile, hyssop, lemongrass, sage, and trumpet vine

Communication Powder

These essential oils are reputed to open communication skills to enable us to get our thoughts across to another person. This powder will make talking easier and help to calm your racing thoughts and tumultuous emotions. Bring your throat chakra into balance while you sleep with this recipe and wake up ready to speak your thoughts clearly and precisely. Therapeutic properties in this blend include antidepressant, tonic, nervine, and sudorific attributes.

Yield: ¼ cup

RECIPE
8 drops geranium oil
4 drops sage oil
3 drops hyssop oil
4 drops vitamin E oil
¼ cup cornstarch

Place the ingredients into a mason jar, stirring well with a whisk. Carefully poke holes into the lid, use this as a shaker, and shake the ingredients into pillowcases or under

sheet areas as needed. You can get a piece of plastic wrap and place it over the jar and under the lid to keep powder from spilling out when not in use. Store in a glass jar or container with a tight-fitting lid in a cool, dark, and dry area for up to 3 months.

Clear the Air

Run this diffuser when you are planning on communicating with others, arguing your side, or trying to get your point across. These essential oils are known for opening the lines of communication and balancing the throat chakra, but more importantly for making it easier for others to listen with an open heart while you are speaking your truth.

Yield: 1 application

RECIPE
6 drops geranium oil
2 drops sage oil
2 drops lavender oil
Water

Follow your directions for using essential oils in your particular brand of diffuser. Ensure that your diffuser does not use heat but runs by vibration, sound waves, or another cold-steam type of process. Choose the essential oils needed for your condition, then add water and oils to the diffuser. Run your diffuser as needed to permeate the air with therapeutic properties and achieve the results you desire.

Tell It to Me Spray

These essential oils are reputed to help you be a better listener and be able to walk in another person's shoes. Open your mind and soul with this blend and receive communication from the universe and those around you. This empathy-inducing blend is helpful when dealing with drama and angst-filled teenagers; these oils will have them listening to you and you listening to them without judgment.

Yield: 2 fluid ounces

RECIPE
3 drops cosmos oil
5 drops hyssop oil

2 drops trumpet vine

1 drop German chamomile oil

3 drops vitamin E oil

1 tablespoon witch hazel

2 fluid ounces water

Add all ingredients to a dark-colored spray bottle. Check for material steadfastness before spraying on fabric. Shake the bottle and spray onto area desired, such as body, hair, home, car, or office. Do not spray into or on open wounds, genitals, eyes, or mucus membranes. Store in a cool, dark area for up to 3 months. Shake well before each use to combine the ingredients.

Communication Bath

Bathe in the essential oils that are said to help you to speak, think, talk, and listen to your utmost ability by healing your throat chakra. Working on the throat chakra is one of the most important gifts you can give to yourself, your friends, and your family. These amazing aromas not only have you feeling like you've spent the day at the spa, but will relax and open the lines of communication between you and those you meet all day.

Yield: 1 application

RECIPE

3 drops hyssop oil

3 drops lemongrass oil

5 drops geranium oil

1 tablespoon carrier oil

1 tablespoon milk (optional for adults, recommended for children)

As you begin to fill the tub with water, pour the chosen essential oils and carrier oil into the running water. Run a warm, not hot, bath. Water that is too hot will cause the essential oils to dissipate. You may add 1 tablespoon of milk to the water; this ensures that the essential oils will not stick to your skin, but will mix with the water. You may soak in the water as long as you are comfortable. Dry your feet well once you get out of the water, as the oils will cause them to be slippery, increasing your chances of falling. Rinse the tub of any remaining oils.

Throat Bath Salts

Not only do the salts and the warm bath water help you to focus on your thoughts, but these essential oils will also help you have the ability to communicate those thoughts to others. While relaxing in this essential oil blend, think about whom you need to talk to, what you need to say, and what you want others to think about your delivery. These oils will help you to achieve that goal while bringing your throat chakra into balance.

Yield: 3 cups

RECIPE
8 drops German chamomile oil
5 drops hyssop oil
5 drops geranium oil
2 tablespoons carrier oil
4 drops vitamin E oil
3 cups bath salts
1 tablespoon milk (optional for adults, recommended for children)

Use any type of salt you prefer: pink Himalayan salt, sea salt, Epsom salts, etc. In a small container, add the essential oils to the desired type of salt. Stir until well blended. Screw lid onto container tightly. Leave mixture in a dark area for 24 hours and then stir mixture again. Run the bathwater. Once the tub is full of water, you can add the milk, and then add ½ cup of the bath salt mixture to bathwater as you get into the tub. You may stay in the tub as long as the temperature is comfortable. Dry your feet well when you get out of the bath, as the oils are slippery and can cause you to fall. Store remainder in a glass jar or container with a tight-fitting lid in a cool, dark area for up to 3 months. These jars make attractive, inexpensive, and healing gifts!

Third Eye Chakra (Ajna)

Located on our forehead, the third eye chakra is our sixth chakra and is where our wisdom, intelligence, and intuition lie. This chakra is responsible for us having an open mind and dealing with thoughts and intuition. To open yourself up to everything the universe has to offer, work with these recipes daily and meditate or pray and you will be on the right path to balancing all of your chakras, becoming increasingly intuitive, and reaching your highest spiritual self. Intellect, awareness, and self-criticisms are developed in the third eye chakra.

Essential Oils

Clary sage, frankincense, lavender, peppermint, rosemary, and spruce

Third Eye Linen Powder

Sharpen your intuition skills while you sleep. Awaken openly to the day when you may need to pay attention to every thought and feeling that you have. Try to remember your dreams and heed any warnings. The therapeutic properties in this blend include sedative, tranquilizing, and antidepressant components.

Yield: ¼ cup

RECIPE

8 drops lavender oil

3 drops clary sage oil

3 drops frankincense oil

4 drops vitamin E oil

¼ cup cornstarch

Place the ingredients into a mason jar, stirring well with a whisk. Carefully poke holes into the lid, use this as a shaker, and shake the ingredients into pillowcases or under sheet areas as needed. You can get a piece of plastic wrap and place it over the jar and under the lid to keep powder from spilling out when not in use. Store in a glass jar or container with a tight-fitting lid in a cool, dark, and dry area for up to 3 months.

Air of Wisdom

Run this in your diffuser to help you to strengthen your third eye chakra by using the essential oils reputed to open your mind, soul, and heart to others. Be open to the gifts you can receive that will help you to grow mentally, spiritually, and physically.

Yield: 1 application

RECIPE
3 drops clary sage oil
2 drops rosemary oil
4 drops lavender oil
Water

Follow your directions for using essential oils in your particular brand of diffuser. Ensure that your diffuser does not use heat but runs by vibration, sound waves, or another cold-steam type of process. Choose the essential oils needed for your condition, then add water and oils to the diffuser. Run your diffuser as needed to permeate the air with therapeutic properties and achieve the results you desire.

Intuition Spray

Use this special spray to tune in to the universe and learn to accept what the universe is offering to you by listening to subtle signs that you would otherwise ignore. The answers are all around you—be open; accept them.

Yield: 2 fluid ounces

RECIPE
8 drops clary sage oil
5 drops peppermint oil
3 drop frankincense oil
3 drops vitamin E oil
1 tablespoon witch hazel
2 fluid ounces water

Add all ingredients to a dark-colored spray bottle. Check for material steadfastness before spraying on fabric. Shake the bottle and spray onto area desired, such as body,

hair, home, car, or office. Do not spray into or on open wounds, genitals, eyes, or mucus membranes. Store in a cool, dark area for up to 3 months. Shake well before each use to combine the ingredients.

Intuition Bath

Bathe yourself in the essential oils that will help you to balance your third eye chakra and develop the skills you need to understand warnings, signs, and blessings from the universe.

Yield: 1 application

RECIPE
5 drops clary sage oil
3 drops lavender oil
2 drops spruce oil
1 tablespoon carrier oil
1 tablespoon milk (optional for adults, recommended for children)

As you begin to fill the tub with water, pour the chosen essential oils and carrier oil into the running water. Run a warm, not hot, bath. Water that is too hot will cause the essential oils to dissipate. You may add 1 tablespoon of milk to the water; this ensures that the essential oils will not stick to your skin, but will mix with the water. You may soak in the water as long as you are comfortable. Dry your feet well once you get out of the water, as the oils will cause them to be slippery, increasing your chances of falling. Rinse the tub of any remaining oils.

Third Eye Bath Salts

These essential oils will help you to balance your third eye chakra and communicate prayers about what you really need in your life. Believe in what you feel and think, and accept the signs that are coming to you from everywhere.

Yield: 3 cups

RECIPE
8 drops clary sage oil
5 drops spruce oil

5 drops frankincense oil

2 tablespoons carrier oil

5 drops vitamin E oil

3 cups bath salts

1 tablespoon milk (optional for adults, recommended for children)

Use any type of salt you prefer: pink Himalayan salt, sea salt, Epsom salts, etc. In a small container, add the essential oils to the desired type of salt. Stir until well blended. Screw lid onto container tightly. Leave mixture in a dark area for 24 hours and then stir mixture again. Run the bathwater. Once the tub is full of water, you can add the milk, and then add ½ cup of the bath salt mixture to bathwater as you get into the tub. You may stay in the tub as long as the temperature is comfortable. Dry your feet well when you get out of the bath, as the oils are slippery and can cause you to fall. Store remainder in a glass jar or container with a tight-fitting lid in a cool, dark area for up to 3 months. These jars make attractive, inexpensive, and healing gifts!

Crown Chakra (Sahasrara)

The seventh chakra is the crown chakra, located at the top of our skull. This chakra is not going to be balanced until all of the other chakras are in balance. The crown chakra is responsible for spirituality, and this chakra needs continual work, for the rest of your life, to keep the soul in balance with the physical aspects of the body. When working with your chakras to bring all aspects of your life into balance, always work on your crown chakra so that you will be in sync with your spirit. Divinity, wisdom, and universal awareness are developed continuously at the crown chakra.

Essential Oils

Angelica, benzoin, frankincense, jasmine, lavender, lotus, myrrh, niaouli, sandalwood, and St. John's wort

Crown Powder

Using the essential oils in this powder as you sleep will enhance knowing that the foundation of everything in the universe is our spirituality. Open your soul to Spirit and listen; you are given what you need.

Yield: ¼ cup

RECIPE

7 drops lavender oil

5 drops niaouli oil

3 drops lotus oil

4 drops vitamin E oil

¼ cup cornstarch

Place the ingredients into a mason jar, stirring well with a whisk. Carefully poke holes into the lid, use this as a shaker, and shake the ingredients into pillowcases or under sheet areas as needed. You can get a piece of plastic wrap and place it over the jar and under the lid to keep powder from spilling out when not in use. Store in a glass jar or container with a tight-fitting lid in a cool, dark, and dry area for up to 3 months.

Balance Mist

The essential oils in this blend will help you to balance your crown chakra, open your spiritual side, and increase your spiritual awareness. You may be drawn to prayer and meditation when this blend is running and balancing all of your chakras.

Yield: 1 application

RECIPE

2 drops lavender oil

3 drops angelica oil

2 drops lotus oil

Water

Follow your directions for using essential oils in your particular brand of diffuser. Ensure that your diffuser does not use heat but runs by vibration, sound waves, or an-

other cold-steam type of process. Choose the essential oils needed for your condition, then add water and oils to the diffuser. Run your diffuser as needed to permeate the air with therapeutic properties and achieve the results you desire.

Chakra-Balancing Spray

I love to spray this as I meditate and pray, and it seriously helps me to focus better and brings my crown chakra into the forefront, thereby helping to balance all of my chakras.

Yield: 2 fluid ounces

RECIPE
7 drops frankincense oil
5 drops myrrh oil
3 drops St. John's wort oil
3 drops vitamin E oil
1 tablespoon witch hazel
2 fluid ounces water

Add all ingredients to a dark-colored spray bottle. Check for material steadfastness before spraying on fabric. Shake the bottle and spray onto area desired, such as body, hair, home, car, or office. Do not spray into or on open wounds, genitals, eyes, or mucus membranes. Store in a cool, dark area for up to 3 months. Shake well before each use to combine the ingredients.

Chakra-Balancing Bath

Every one of these essential oils is used in religious and sacred rituals the world over. You too can use this special blend to enhance your spiritual journey, open your soul, and accept what is being given to you every second of every day.

Yield: 1 application

RECIPE
3 drops sandalwood oil
4 drops jasmine oil

4 drops angelica oil

2 drops niaouli oil

1 tablespoon carrier oil

1 tablespoon milk (optional for adults, recommended for children)

As you begin to fill the tub with water, pour the chosen essential oils and carrier oil into the running water. Run a warm, not hot, bath. Water that is too hot will cause the essential oils to dissipate. You may add 1 tablespoon of milk to the water; this ensures that the essential oils will not stick to your skin, but will mix with the water. You may soak in the water as long as you are comfortable. Dry your feet well once you get out of the water, as the oils will cause them to be slippery, increasing your chances of falling. Rinse the tub of any remaining oils.

Crown Bath Salts

These essential oils will open the windows of your soul as you pray, meditate, and relax in a calming, soothing, purifying, and cleansing bath. Believe in what you want, need, and ask for, and it will come to you.

Yield: 3 cups

RECIPE

8 drops angelica oil

5 drops niaouli oil

5 drops myrrh oil

2 tablespoons carrier oil

4 drops vitamin E oil

3 cups salts

1 tablespoon milk (optional for adults, recommended for children)

Use any type of salt you prefer: pink Himalayan salt, sea salt, Epsom salts, etc. In a small container, add the essential oils to the desired type of salt. Stir until well blended. Screw lid onto container tightly. Leave mixture in a dark area for 24 hours and then stir mixture again. Run the bathwater. Once the tub is full of water, you can add the milk, and then add ½ cup of the bath salt mixture to bathwater as you get into the tub. You may stay in the tub as long as the temperature is comfortable. Dry your feet well when you get out of the bath, as the oils are slippery and can cause you to fall. Store remainder in a glass jar or container with a tight-fitting lid in a cool, dark area for up to 3 months. These jars make attractive, inexpensive, and healing gifts!

Introduction to Doshas

Doshas are the three energies that each and every person has that influence their physical, mental, and spiritual selves. The doshas are often out of balance, and a person may have one dosha that is influencing their lives in a negative manner such as causing illness, depression, disease, or anxiety. In most of the Far Eastern countries, when a person is ill, the doshas are the first thing about a person to be determined in order to evaluate the course of treatment that will balance the doshas and lead that person to good health. The doshas can be affected by diet, exercise, meditation, attitude, living environment, and chemical factors, to name a few. There are many ways to balance out the doshas so that a person is at their optimal best. Essential oils can play a big part in balancing your dosha and helping you to achieve the mental, physical, and spiritual health you desire.

The doshas are a type of personality classification and are divided mainly into three categories: vata, pitta, and kapha. This ancient Ayurvedic system of dividing people's personalities and energies into classifications of doshas is helpful on so many levels. Knowing that vatas get one type of disease, kaphas get another, and pittas get totally different illnesses helps us to control all facets of our lives by not letting our doshas get out of balance, enabling us to stave off these particular diseases.

Once a particular dosha is discovered to be prominent in yourself, you can work through diet, herbs, yoga, meditation, various therapies, and essential oils to lower the dominant dosha and raise the other doshas to bring balance. Balancing the doshas is the number one way of preventing the prevalent diseases associated with your dosha. We are all born with one, or sometimes two, doshas dominating our personalities, spirituality, mentality, and physicality. Learning to lower our dominant dosha and bring balance to our doshas is at the forefront of all Ayurvedic healing.

Many times you can look at a person, watch them for several minutes, and know what type of dosha is foremost in their constitutional makeup. Learning about reducing and balancing your doshas can add years to your life, and make the life you live happier and healthier.

Everyone has all three doshas that make up their inner selves. But balancing out the doshas so that one of them is not extremely dominant is the aim of Ayurvedic teaching and healing. Knowing that someone is a kapha, pitta, or vata can give them an edge when looking at long-term health care and happiness. Understanding that you are a kapha and that you are *way* too sedentary and are prone to heart disease and obesity can help you learn to add more vata to your life and become more active, eat healthier, and use the essential oils known for lowering your kapha and raising your pitta and vata levels. It's all about balance.

Researching and learning about the doshas can have such a huge impact on people and on their lives, mentally, spiritually, and physically. In this section I give some examples of how the doshas can cause certain emotions in people and provide lists of essential oils that can be used to reduce that dominant dosha and bring them more into balance. This, in turn, staves off illness in many forms, and helps to heal illnesses already present.

There are many websites devoted to testing your doshas for free. The tests are simply a list of questions, and the scores can determine which dosha, or doshas, are prominent in your characteristics. It's fun and easy. The insight you can gain into yourself and your family is astonishing. Take two or three of the online free tests and see if they all come up with the same dosha. Be honest with your answers; this can sometimes be difficult. Discovering which doshas are out of balance in a household family member can be quite eye-opening and give you answers as to why they act the way that they do. Knowing that you can massage them with a certain oil or diffuse other oils to help balance the doshas that have gotten out of control in certain family members can be a powerful tool in the road to harmony.

You will be surprised when you can determine what dosha some of your older relatives are and notice that they really do have the diseases that are associated with that particular dosha. Then you will be armed with numerous ways to lower their prominent dosha, bring their doshas into balance, and drastically reduce their chances of ending up with many diseases and health issues related to their doshas being out of balance. To be forewarned is to be forearmed.

Here is a list of characteristics that usually apply to a particular dosha. Keep count of all that apply to you, then see which dosha you have the most of and which you have the least of. Try to lower the dosha that is too high, and raise the dosha that is too low. If you have close to the same number of checks in all three doshas, then you are a well-balanced person.

Vata

- Fast talker
- Fast walker
- Usually a leader
- Thin body type
- Light sleeper
- Digestive issues
- Frizzy hair
- Dry skin
- Usually anxious or fearful
- Always cold
- Impulsive spending
- Hard worker
- Joint and muscle pain

Kapha

- Large body frame
- Overweight
- Slow activity level
- Long-lasting friendships
- Calm personality
- Does not like drama
- Good with finances
- Slow speech

- Sleeps easily
- Thick hair
- Dislikes humid weather
- Slow digestion
- Sinus issues

Pitta

- Medium body type
- Average sleep
- Light eyes
- Hates heat
- Intense emotions
- Quick to anger/laughter
- Good digestion
- Intelligent
- Goal oriented
- Occasionally spends money frivolously
- Workaholic
- Argues and wins
- Light or red hair

Kapha

A person with a dominant kapha is likely to be slow-paced, non-judgmental, relaxed, calm, loving, understanding, and overweight. Kaphas tend to have congestion and sinus issues. Essential oils can be used to give a Kapha person some energy, lower their kapha dosha, and get them moving. Kaphas can keep secrets, and other people trust them. While kaphas tend to have positive personalities, they tend to need much more exercise and movements than they typically get for their health. Some of these recipes are chock-full of energy-inducing oils. Kaphas are prone to heart and high blood pressure illnesses, diseases brought on by obesity, and knee and joint pain. These recipes can help to reduce those illnesses by promoting activity and calm.

Essential Oils

Anise, basil, bay laurel, bergamot, black pepper, camphor, cardamom, cinnamon, clary sage, clove, cypress, eucalyptus, grapefruit, hyssop, jasmine, juniper, lavender, lemon, lemongrass, lime, marjoram, myrrh, neroli, petitgrain, rose, rosemary, sweet orange, and yarrow

Kapha Bath Salts

To increase your vata and pitta, soak in these essential oils and feel your energy level rising. Reducing your kapha dosha will help you to feel more energetic, thereby reducing your weight and getting your heart and blood pumping properly.

Yield: 3 cups

RECIPE
5 drops cardamom oil
5 drops clary sage oil
7 drops orange oil
3 drops marjoram oil
2 tablespoons carrier oil
5 drops vitamin E oil
3 cups salts
1 tablespoon milk (optional for adults, recommended for children)

Use any type of salt you prefer: pink Himalayan salt, sea salt, Epsom salts, etc. In a small container, add the essential oils to the desired type of salt. Stir until well blended. Screw lid onto container tightly. Leave mixture in a dark area for 24 hours and then stir mixture again. Run the bathwater. Once the tub is full of water, you can add the milk, and then add ½ cup of the bath salt mixture to bathwater as you get into the tub. You may stay in the tub as long as the temperature is comfortable. Dry your feet well when you get out of the bath, as the oils are slippery and can cause you

to fall. Store remainder in a glass jar or container with a tight-fitting lid in a cool, dark area for up to 3 months. These jars make attractive, inexpensive, and healing gifts!

Bring Down That Kapha Spray

When you start feeling sluggish and too full of mucus, use this spray to get you up and going. Decongesting and energizing therapeutic properties abound in this blend. This recipe will bring down that mucus-inducing kapha dosha and heighten your vata and pitta doshas.

Yield: 2 fluid ounces

RECIPE

4 drops anise oil

3 drops lemongrass oil

2 drops eucalyptus oil

1 drop rosemary oil

2 drops bay laurel oil

1 drop yarrow oil

1 tablespoon witch hazel

2 fluid ounces water

Add all ingredients to a dark-colored spray bottle. Check for material steadfastness before spraying on fabric. Shake the bottle and spray onto area desired, such as body, hair, home, car, or office. Do not spray into or on open wounds, genitals, eyes, or mucus membranes. Store in a cool, dark area for up to 3 months. Shake well before each use to combine the ingredients.

Cut the Kapha Air

These are the essential oils that are reported to bring down your kapha and bring your doshas into balance. This general kapha-reducing diffuser will help to motivate you to get out of your chair, take a walk, and start a project with their energizing properties and focusing aromas.

Yield: 1 application

RECIPE
2 drops basil oil
3 drops sweet orange oil
2 drops ginger oil
3 drops rose oil
Water

Follow your directions for using essential oils in your particular brand of diffuser. Ensure that your diffuser does not use heat but runs by vibration, sound waves, or another cold-steam type of process. Choose the essential oils needed for your condition, then add water and oils to the diffuser. Run your diffuser as needed to permeate the air with therapeutic properties and achieve the results you desire.

Kapha-Reducing Bath

Relaxing seems to be the trait of kaphas, but after this bath, you will have the energy to go, go, go! Kaphas need to find ways to increase their motivation as much as possible in order to stave off those kapha illnesses such as high blood pressure and heart disease.

Yield: 1 application

RECIPE
3 drops rose oil
2 drops neroli oil
2 drops grapefruit oil
1 drop myrrh oil
4 drops petitgrain oil
1 tablespoon carrier oil
1 tablespoon milk (optional for adults, recommended for children)

As you begin to fill the tub with water, pour the chosen essential oils and carrier oil into the running water. Run a warm, not hot, bath. Water that is too hot will cause the essential oils to dissipate. You may add 1 tablespoon of milk to the water; this ensures that the essential oils will not stick to your skin, but will mix with the water. You may soak in the water as long as you are comfortable. Dry your feet well once you get out of the water, as the oils will cause them to be slippery, increasing your chances of falling. Rinse the tub of any remaining oils.

For Kaphas Only Inhaler

Clear out the kapha mucus and get going with this inhale. These essential oils are great for that stuffy head that kaphas seem to experience quite often. The therapeutic properties are expectorant and decongestant agents to help you breathe again.

Yield: 1 application

RECIPE
1 drop lavender oil

or

1 drop rose oil

or

1 drop lemon oil

Choose your essential oil and apply to the palm of your hand, an oil inhaler, or a tissue. Bring the essential oils close to your nostrils and inhale the aroma deeply. You can cover one nostril at a time with your thumb and, if you prefer, alternate nostrils. This process sends the properties straight to your brain and the effects are immediate. You can complete this process 3–4 times daily.

Rub That Kapha Away

This is a blend of essential oils that are specifically designed to reduce the kapha dosha and increase the vata and pitta to get you energized and feeling excited about life. Shake off that kapha lethargy and increase those energetic and airy vata traits.

Yield: 2 tablespoons

RECIPE
4 drops jasmine oil
2 drops bergamot oil

> 3 drops clary sage oil
>
> 1 drop cardamom oil
>
> 3 drops vitamin E oil
>
> 2 tablespoons carrier oil

Pour the essential oils, carrier oil, and any remaining ingredients into a small glass container, bowl, or jar. Swirl or whisk to mix the ingredients and apply lightly to the area desired, such as pressure points, neck, soles of feet, temples, or chest. Keep essential oil mixture away from open wounds, mucus membranes, genitals, eyes, and sensitive areas. Repeat application as needed, usually 2–3 times daily. You may cover area with linen or cloth to protect clothing and furniture. Store unused portion in a glass jar or container with a tight-fitting lid in a cool, dark area for up to 3 months.

Kapha-Reducing Linen Powder

Sleep on this powder all night long and wake up with renewed vigor and energy. These oils will help impart the desire and focus you need to begin an exercise / movement routine after a great night's sleep. Decrease those kapha tendencies with the essential oils in this recipe.

Yield: ¼ cup

RECIPE

5 drops jasmine oil

5 drops rose oil

5 drops lavender oil

4 drops vitamin E oil

¼ cup cornstarch

Place the ingredients into a mason jar, stirring well with a whisk. Carefully poke holes into the lid, use this as a shaker, and shake the ingredients into pillowcases or under sheet areas as needed. You can get a piece of plastic wrap and place it over the jar and under the lid to keep powder from spilling out when not in use. Store in a glass jar or container with a tight-fitting lid in a cool, dark, and dry area for up to 3 months.

Vata

Quick thinkers, talkers, and walkers. Vatas tend to hate cold weather and have dry hair and skin. Essential oils can assist with moistening the skin of the vata person among many other vata-reducing properties. Vatas are prone to extreme mood changes. Vatas are usually leaders; some say it's because they are too quick to follow anyone! Essential oils can balance the moods of the vata, and calm a vata down to normal speed when they are running themselves thin. Bringing the vata down to earth can be challenging, as they do tend to go from one extreme to the other. Vatas are nervous, fearful, and have extreme anxiety. These essential oils can help with not only slowing you down, but doing it with a happy heart, mind, and soul. Vatas usually end up with painful illnesses such as various types of arthritis, muscle, joint, back, and tendon pain.

Essential Oils

Bay laurel, bergamot, camphor, cardamom, chamomile, cinnamon, clary sage, eucalyptus, frankincense, ginger, jasmine, lavender, lemongrass, myrrh, neroli, patchouli, sandalwood, sesame, sweet orange, tangerine, thyme, vanilla, vetiver, and ylang-ylang

Vata Bath Salts

If you can get a vata to slow down long enough to take a leisurely bath instead of a quick shower, this is the recipe for them. These essential oils will help a vata to not want to run themselves to death, but to slow down a little and enjoy life. These oils help to eliminate fear and anxiety as well, which are huge vata traits. A few of the therapeutic properties in this recipe include sudorific, tonic, sedative, nervine, and aphrodisiac components.

Yield: 3 cups

RECIPE
5 drops tangerine oil
5 drops ginger oil
5 drops neroli oil
5 drops lemongrass oil

5 drops vitamin E oil

2 tablespoons carrier oil

3 cups salts

1 tablespoon milk (optional for adults, recommended for children)

Use any type of salt you prefer: pink Himalayan salt, sea salt, Epsom salts, etc. In a small container, add the essential oils to the desired type of salt. Stir until well blended. Screw lid onto container tightly. Leave mixture in a dark area for 24 hours and then stir mixture again. Run the bathwater. Once the tub is full of water, you can add the milk, and then add ½ cup of the bath salt mixture to bathwater as you get into the tub. These jars make attractive, inexpensive, and healing gifts! Store remainder in a glass jar or container with a tight-fitting lid in a cool, dark area for up to 3 months.

Mellow Me Out Spray

The essential oils in this spray are perfect for the vata person. Vatas are so stressed at all times and full of anxiety. These oils help to ground them with mellowing properties. The essential oils are calming, peaceful, and will help a vata to increase their kapha and pitta doshas.

Yield: 2 fluid ounces

RECIPE

3 drops lavender oil

3 drops vetiver oil

2 drops ylang-ylang oil

2 drops clary sage oil

1 drop bay laurel oil

3 drops vitamin E oil

1 tablespoon witch hazel

2 fluid ounces water

Add all ingredients to a dark-colored spray bottle. Check for material steadfastness before spraying on fabric. Shake the bottle and spray onto area desired, such as body, hair, home, car, or office. Do not spray into or on open wounds, genitals, eyes, or mucus membranes. Store in a cool, dark area for up to 3 months. Shake well before each use to combine the ingredients.

Vata Is Air

Vatas are associated with the "air" signs, and getting grounded is a great way to reduce the vata dosha. Bring balance to your doshas with this diffuse of essential oils specifically designed to reduce vata and increase the pitta and kapha. This is the perfect diffuser to run if you or someone visiting you is very anxious or nervous. This blend has grounding and calming therapeutic properties.

Yield: 1 application

RECIPE
3 drops neroli oil
2 drops frankincense oil
2 drops ginger oil
1 drop jasmine oil
Water

Follow your directions for using essential oils in your particular brand of diffuser. Ensure that your diffuser does not use heat but runs by vibration, sound waves, or another cold-steam type of process. Choose the essential oils needed for your condition, then add water and oils to the diffuser. Run your diffuser as needed to permeate the air with therapeutic properties and achieve the results you desire.

Anxiety-Lessening Bath

Vatas are prone to anxiety, worrying, and needless fidgeting. The essential oils in this bath will force them to slow down, relax, and enjoy the good things in life, not rush it. Vatas do need to chill a bit, quit overanalyzing everything, and stop sweating the small stuff. Vatas can also use this recipe to increase their pitta and kapha elements in order to curb their impulsivity, reckless spending, and hyper traits. These sedative, calming, and grounding properties work well to reduce vata tendencies.

Yield: 1 application

RECIPE
3 drops bay laurel oil
3 drops neroli oil
3 drops mandarin oil
2 drops lemongrass oil
1 drop vetiver oil
1 tablespoon carrier oil
1 tablespoon milk (optional for adults, recommended for children)

As you begin to fill the tub with water, pour the chosen essential oils and carrier oil into the running water. Run a warm, not hot, bath. Water that is too hot will cause the essential oils to dissipate. You may add 1 tablespoon of milk to the water; this ensures that the essential oils will not stick to your skin, but will mix with the water. You may soak in the water as long as you are comfortable. Dry your feet well once you get out of the water, as the oils will cause them to be slippery, increasing your chances of falling. Rinse the tub of any remaining oils.

For Vatas Only

These calming essential oils are perfect for one who has too much vata. Carry vials with you and use it whenever you find your thoughts racing and are unable to concentrate on the task at hand. Vatas are like butterflies flitting from one thing to another, and they often need grounding several times a day. These essential oils are known to increase the pitta and kapha in a person, while providing grounding agents with just a tiny smell of the oils.

Yield: 1 application

RECIPE
1 drop vetiver oil
or
1 drop frankincense oil
or
1 drop neroli oil

Choose your essential oil and apply to the palm of your hand, an oil inhaler, or a tissue. Bring the essential oils close to your nostrils and inhale the aroma deeply. You can cover one nostril at a time with your thumb and, if you prefer, alternate nostrils. This process sends the properties straight to your brain and the effects are immediate. You can complete this process 3–4 times daily.

Zen Rub

Bring your doshas into balance with this rub that uses essential oils that will quell the vata in you and bring your kapha and pitta a little higher. Ground yourself while getting all of the benefits of tons of therapeutic properties inherent in this blend, such as sedative, calming, and aphrodisiac elements.

Yield: 2–6 applications

RECIPE
3 drops tangerine oil
1 drop vanilla oil
2 drops vetiver oil
2 drops myrrh oil
3 drops vitamin E oil
1 tablespoon carrier oil

Pour the essential oils, carrier oil, and any remaining ingredients into a small glass container, bowl, or jar. Swirl or whisk to mix the ingredients and apply lightly to the area desired, such as pressure points, neck, soles of feet, temples, or chest. Keep essential oil mixture away from open wounds, mucus membranes, genitals, eyes, and sensitive areas. Repeat application as needed, usually 2–3 times daily. You may cover area with linen or cloth to protect clothing and furniture. Store unused portion in a glass jar or container with a tight-fitting lid in a cool, dark area for up to 3 months.

Vata Linen Powder

Go to bed anxious and worried, and then wake up a calmer and more peaceful person after using this essential oil and powder mixture. Increase your kapha and pitta and reduce your vata with this blend by sleeping on the calming properties used here.

Yield: ¼ cup

RECIPE

4 drops vetiver oil

3 drops vanilla oil

2 drops rosewood oil

1 drop sandalwood oil

4 drops myrrh oil

4 drops vitamin E oil

¼ cup cornstarch

Place the ingredients into a mason jar, stirring well with a whisk. Carefully poke holes into the lid, use this as a shaker, and shake the ingredients into pillowcases or under sheet areas as needed. You can get a piece of plastic wrap and place it over the jar and under the lid to keep powder from spilling out when not in use. Store in a glass jar or container with a tight-fitting lid in a cool, dark, and dry area for up to 3 months.

Pitta

Pittas have the ability to be great public speakers. They don't like hot weather and perspire heavily. Pittas are quick to anger and quick to laugh. They tend to have skin issues, such as eczema or rashes, when under stress. Pittas enjoy romance, love, and laughter. Pittas do need some mellowing, usually not physically but emotionally. These balancing essential oils will bring in a little kapha and vata to balance the pitta. Pittas are great at arguing, holding grudges, bringing up every little thing from the past, and harboring resentment. Calming essential oils can help pittas learn to just "let go." These traits cause pittas to end up suffering from high blood pressure, strokes, and other adrenaline-packed illnesses. Balancing out the pitta dosha is as easy as adding a few things to the diet, removing a few things, using the correct herbs and essential oils, and moving on a path to a more spiritual place in their lives.

Essential Oils

Birch, coriander, fennel, lavender, lemon balm (melissa), lime, mandarin, myrtle, peppermint, petitgrain, spearmint, sunflower, tangerine, tea tree, wintergreen, and yarrow

Let It Go Bath Salts

Pittas are quick to anger, and these bath salts have essential oils that are reputed to bring that anger down and replace it with some mood-balancing contemplation. So if you feel yourself going over the top about something trivial... slow it down with this blend. The therapeutic properties in this blend include aphrodisiac, sedative, antidepressant, and nervine agents.

Yield: 3 cups

RECIPE
5 drops coriander oil
5 drops petitgrain oil
5 drops myrtle oil
5 drops tangerine oil
2 tablespoons carrier oil
5 drops vitamin E oil
3 cups salts
1 tablespoon milk (optional for adults, recommended for children)

Use any type of salt you prefer: pink Himalayan salt, sea salt, Epsom salts, etc. In a small container, add the essential oils to the desired type of salt. Stir until well blended. Screw lid onto container tightly. Leave mixture in a dark area for 24 hours and then stir mixture again. Run the bathwater. Once the tub is full of water, you can add the milk, and then add ½ cup of the bath salt mixture to bathwater as you get into the tub. You may stay in the tub as long as the temperature is comfortable. Dry your feet well when you get out of the bath, as the oils are slippery and can cause you to fall. Store remainder in a glass jar or container with a tight-fitting lid in a cool, dark area for up to 3 months. These jars make attractive, inexpensive, and healing gifts!

Pitta Cooling Spray

Pittas are hot all the time. Carry this spray with you and cool yourself down in a flash with these cooling essential oils. This is a refreshing bottle of spray that you can carry in your purse, leave at the office, or take on vacation. Reduce that pitta heat and cool down your emotions as well as your body with this blend.

Yield: 2 fluid ounces

RECIPE

4 drops spearmint oil

4 drops peppermint oil

3 drops lemon balm oil (melissa oil)

1 tablespoon witch hazel

2 fluid ounces water

Add all ingredients to a dark-colored spray bottle. Check for material steadfastness before spraying on fabric. Shake the bottle and spray onto area desired, such as body, hair, home, car, or office. Do not spray into or on open wounds, genitals, eyes, or mucus membranes. Store in a cool, dark area for up to 3 months. Shake well before each use to combine the ingredients.

Air Conditioner Diffuser

This diffuser recipe is known as "God's little air conditioner." The essential oils used in this recipe are known to cool down the air and bring relief to that pitta who is always burning up!

Yield: 1 application

RECIPE

3 drops peppermint oil

3 drops mandarin oil

2 drops lime oil

1 drop myrtle oil

Water

Follow your directions for using essential oils in your particular brand of diffuser. Ensure that your diffuser does not use heat but runs by vibration, sound waves, or another cold-steam type of process. Choose the essential oils needed for your condition, then add water and oils to the diffuser. Run your diffuser as needed to permeate the air with therapeutic properties and achieve the results you desire.

Pitta-Balancing Bath

Reduce that pitta and increase your vata and kapha with this recipe that uses essential oils to balance your doshas. The essential oils in this blend will give you uplifted feelings, assuage any anger, and provide you with energy-inducing momentum.

Yield: 1 application

RECIPE
3 drops coriander oil
1 drop fennel oil
3 drops myrtle oil
3 drops petitgrain oil
2 drops tea tree (melaleuca) oil
1 tablespoon carrier oil
1 tablespoon milk (optional for adults, recommended for children)

As you begin to fill the tub with water, pour the chosen essential oils and carrier oil into the running water. Run a warm, not hot, bath. Water that is too hot will cause the essential oils to dissipate. You may add 1 tablespoon of milk to the water; this ensures that the essential oils will not stick to your skin, but will mix with the water. You may soak in the water as long as you are comfortable. Dry your feet well once you get out of the water, as the oils will cause them to be slippery, increasing your chances of falling. Rinse the tub of any remaining oils.

For Pittas Only Inhaler

When needing to bring your emotions under control, take a whiff of these essential oils. Pittas tend to let their emotions overrule them. These oils will bring you back to earth and help to bring you balance with the calming properties and the grounding quality of these oils.

Yield: 1 application

RECIPE
1 drop peppermint oil

or

1 drop spearmint oil

Choose your essential oil and apply to the palm of your hand, an oil inhaler, or a tissue. Bring the essential oils close to your nostrils and inhale the aroma deeply. You can cover one nostril at a time with your thumb and, if you prefer, alternate nostrils. This process sends the properties straight to your brain and the effects are immediate. You can complete this process 3–4 times daily.

Pitta-Balancing Rub

The essential oils in this recipe are known to bring the doshas into balance for a pitta by raising the vata and kapha. The grounding qualities of these oils keep the emotions under control and promote a sense of well-being.

Yield: 1 fluid ounce

RECIPE
3 drops mandarin oil
3 drops yarrow oil
1 drop fennel oil
1 drop tea tree (melaleuca) oil
3 drops vitamin E oil
1 fluid ounce carrier oil

Pour the essential oils, carrier oil, and any remaining ingredients into a small glass container, bowl, or jar. Swirl or whisk to mix the ingredients and apply lightly to the area desired, such as pressure points, neck, soles of feet, temples, or chest. Keep essential oil mixture away from open wounds, mucus membranes, genitals, eyes, and sensitive areas. Repeat application as needed, usually 2–3 times daily. You may cover area with linen or cloth to protect clothing and furniture. Store unused portion in a glass jar or container with a tight-fitting lid in a cool, dark area for up to 3 months.

Cool Sleep Linen Powder

The essential oils in this recipe have cooling properties and can give a pitta a nice, cool night's sleep and assist in keeping their anxiety, anger, and emotions under control. These oils have cooling, sedative, grounding, antidepressant, nervine, and aromatic properties to bring calm and peace to a pitta in a state of emotional turmoil.

Yield: ¼ cup

RECIPE
5 drops mandarin oil
3 drops petitgrain oil
2 drops spearmint oil
4 drops vitamin E oil
¼ cup cornstarch

Place the ingredients into a mason jar, stirring well with a whisk. Carefully poke holes into the lid, use this as a shaker, and shake the ingredients into pillowcases or under sheet areas as needed. You can get a piece of plastic wrap and place it over the jar and under the lid to keep powder from spilling out when not in use. Store in a glass jar or container with a tight-fitting lid in a cool, dark, and dry area for up to 3 months.

CHAPTER 3
Recipes for Conditions

*N*ow that we've covered how to use essential oils for the chakras and doshas, we will move on to the main portion of the book. Here begins the lists of recipes for conditions, emotions, needs, desires, then, finally, devotions. Throughout history, essential oils, herbs, and various concoctions from plants, flowers, and trees have been used to increase or decrease matters of the mind and spirit. I have researched ancient and new scientific findings to bring to you the essential oils and the recipes that have worked in the past for people and continue to work today.

Under each condition is a list of essential oils that have been used for that particular need. If you do not have an essential oil listed in a certain recipe, then you can substitute an essential oil that you do have from the list. I have tried to simplify the usage of essential oils so that you can develop your own recipes using the basic formats in this book.

Learning to use essential oils can be one of the most beneficial practices you can use to increase your chances of living a longer, happier, and healthier life. Have fun with the following recipes, and incorporate your own ideas when using essential oils. I hope that you have as much fun, experience as much healing, and grow by as many leaps and bounds as I have through the pages of these recipes.

Addictions

Addictions can be mental, physical, and/or emotional. The body and brain become used to a particular substance or behavior and then disregards the consequences of abusing that certain substance. One can overcome addictions through willpower, substituting healthy alternatives, or with medical intervention. Withdrawing from certain addictions, such as medications, can be potentially fatal. Check with your physician to ensure withdrawing from the substance or behavior will not produce any ill effects or that the consequences can be controlled. Medical intervention is often necessary to withdraw from a particular substance. Essential oils can vastly reduce the side effects of withdrawing from addictions.

Essential Oils

Basil, bergamot, black pepper, cilantro, cinnamon, clary sage, clove, Damask rose, grapefruit, helichrysum, jasmine, juniper, melissa, peppermint, sandalwood, wild orange, white fir, and ylang-ylang

Peaceful Pillow Powder

This recipe is mainly used for lulling a person into a peaceful sleep rather than having them lie awake and obsess over their addiction. Focusing on cravings is the last thing you want to do when trying to overcome an addiction. The essential oils in this recipe contain the following compounds: aperient, carminative, digestive, anticonvulsive, antidepressant, emenagogue, euphoric, nervine, sedative, and an aphrodisiac.

Yield: ¾ cup

RECIPE
3 drops Damask rose oil
3 drops grapefruit oil
3 drops clary sage oil
¼ cup cornstarch
4 drops vitamin E oil

Place the ingredients into a mason jar, stirring well with a whisk. Carefully poke holes into the lid, use this as a shaker, and shake the ingredients into pillowcases or under

sheet areas as needed. You can get a piece of plastic wrap and place it over the jar and under the lid to keep powder from spilling out when not in use. Store in a glass jar or container with a tight-fitting lid in a cool, dark area for up to 3 months.

Breathe

When you are trying to break an addiction, this recipe is one you can take with you anywhere. Carry a small vial in your car or purse, and when the urges are strong, take a whiff of this to calm you down and let it all go. The essential oils in this recipe impart beneficial elements to the nasal receptors such as analgesic, anti-inflammatory, aphrodisiac, stimulating, sudorific, nervine, and antispasmodic components.

Yield: 1 application

RECIPE
2 drops clove oil

or

2 drops peppermint oil

Choose your essential oil and apply to the palm of your hand, an oil inhaler, or a tissue. Bring the essential oils close to your nostrils and inhale the aroma deeply. You can cover one nostril at a time with your thumb and, if you prefer, alternate nostrils. This process sends the properties straight to your brain and the effects are immediate. You can complete this process 3–4 times daily.

Fresh, Fresh Air

This mixture is perfect for calming a person and helping them to have a better outlook on life and their issues. This is a happy, joyful blend of aromas that will take your mind off your cravings and have you thinking about a brighter future without harmful substances. Therapeutic properties in these essential oils are antidepressant, disinfectant, stimulant, and tonic.

Yield: 1 application

RECIPE
2 drops grapefruit oil
2 drops clary sage oil

2 drops jasmine oil

Water

Follow your directions for using essential oils in your particular brand of diffuser. Ensure that your diffuser does not use heat but runs by vibration, sound waves, or another cold-steam type of process. Choose the essential oils needed for your condition, then add water and oils to the diffuser. Run your diffuser as needed to permeate the air with therapeutic properties and achieve the results you desire.

Bathe It All Away

Such a wonderful aroma is imparted from this bath mixture. You won't want to leave the tub. These healing, calming essential oils will aid you in the ability to quit focusing on the negative and start focusing on the positive in life. The advantageous essential oils in this recipe contain antidepressant, aphrodisiac, depurative, nervine, antiseptic, and sedative properties.

Yield: 1 application

RECIPE

3 drops Damask rose oil

4 drops juniper oil

7 drops jasmine oil

1 tablespoon carrier oil

1 tablespoon milk (optional for adults, recommended for children)

As you begin to fill the tub with water, pour the chosen essential oils and carrier oil into the running water. Run a warm, not hot, bath. Water that is too hot will cause the essential oils to dissipate. You may add 1 tablespoon of milk to the water; this ensures that the essential oils will not stick to your skin, but will mix with the water. You may soak in the water as long as you are comfortable. Dry your feet well once you get out of the water, as the oils will cause them to be slippery, increasing your chances of falling. Rinse the tub of any remaining oils.

End the Cravings Massage

This massage oil is perfect for energizing a person and lifting them out of a funk. These essential oils will get you ready to face another day and with a smile, banishing the negative effects of withdrawal. The uplifting properties in these essential oils are antioxidant, cooling, stimulating, invigorating, and nervine agents.

Yield: 2 tablespoons

RECIPE
1 drop cinnamon oil
1 drop cilantro oil
2 drops peppermint oil
2 tablespoons carrier oil

Pour the essential oils and the carrier oil into a small glass container, bowl, or jar. Swirl to mix the ingredients and use to lightly massage the area desired such as neck, temples, soles of feet, back, and/or chest. Keep essential oil mixture away from open wounds, mucus membranes, genitals, eyes, and sensitive areas. Repeat application as needed. Store unused portion in a glass jar or container with a tight-fitting lid in a cool, dark area for up to 3 months.

Peaceful Bath Salts

I absolutely love bath salts. I feel that bath salts can get me squeaky clean and heal any wounds, and the essential oils cure what ails me. Not only will your skin feel great, your mood will lift and so will your spirits. Wonderful properties are contained within these essential oils such as antirheumatic, antitoxic, astringent, circulatory stimulant, sudorific, depurative, stimulating, vulnerary, and rubefacient.

Yield: 3 cups

RECIPE
5 drops clary sage oil
5 drops juniper oil
5 drops grapefruit oil

3 cups salts

2 tablespoons carrier oil

1 tablespoon milk (optional for adults, recommended for children)

Use any type of salt you prefer: pink Himalayan salt, sea salt, Epsom salts, etc. In a small container, add the essential oils to the desired type of salt. Stir until the essential oil and salt mixture is well blended. Screw lid onto container tightly. Leave mixture in a dark area for 24 hours and then stir mixture again. Run the bathwater. Once the tub is full of water, you can add the milk, and then add ½ cup of the bath salt mixture to bathwater as you get into the tub. These jars make attractive, inexpensive, and healing gifts! Store in cool, dark area in a glass jar or container with a tight-fitting lid for up to 3 months.

Bipolar

Bipolar is a mental illness characterized by bouts of mania followed by equally devastating bouts of depression. Many pharmaceuticals are available today to assist people with managing their mood swings. Some believe that this condition is hereditary as usually more than one person in a family suffers from bipolar disorder. Various therapies have proven to be beneficial to numerous people suffering from bipolar-related illnesses.

Essential oils

Basil, clary sage, cinnamon, frankincense, lavender, melissa, peppermint, rosemary, spearmint, and vetiver

Mood Controlling Massage

This massage is great for leveling out a person's moods. Whether you are currently manic or depressed, this essential oil blend is good for bringing one to balance and letting you be the master of your moods. These oils contain curative properties, including antidepressant, euphoric, hypotensive, nervine, and sedative properties.

Yield: 2–4 applications

RECIPE

2 drops melissa oil

2 drops frankincense oil

1 drop clary sage oil

1 tablespoon carrier oil

3 drops vitamin E oil

See directions on page 19 or 77.

Calming Inhale

This aroma is reported to level out the hormones and balance the thought processes. The mood-calming properties of these oils are antidepressant, restorative, sedative, and tonic agents.

Yield: 1 application

RECIPE

1 drop lavender oil

1 drop melissa oil

Choose your essential oil and apply to the palm of your hand, an oil inhaler, or a tissue. Bring the essential oils close to your nostrils and inhale the aroma deeply. You can cover one nostril at a time with your thumb and, if you prefer, alternate nostrils. This process sends the properties straight to your brain and the effects are immediate. You can complete this procedure 3–4 times daily.

Revitalizing Bath Salts

Bring a sense of calm, relaxation, and happiness to the brain with this blend. These essential oils are known for their ability to bring soul, mind, and body into harmony with their antidepressant, sedative, and restorative properties. Not to mention you get to relax in a calming salt bath!

Yield: 3 cups

RECIPE

7 drops clary sage oil

7 drops vetiver oil

7 drops lavender oil

3 cups salts

1 tablespoon carrier oil

1 tablespoon milk (optional for adults, recommended for children)

Use any type of salt you prefer: pink Himalayan salt, sea salt, Epsom salts, Etc. In a small container, add the essential oils to the desired type of salt. Stir until well blended. Screw lid onto container tightly. Leave mixture in a dark area for 24 hours and then stir mixture again. Run the bathwater. Once the tub is full of water, you can add the milk, and then add ½ cup of the bath salt mixture to bathwater as you get into the tub. You may stay in the tub as long as the temperature is comfortable. Dry your feet well when you get out of the bath, as the oils are slippery and can cause you to fall. Store remainder in a glass jar or container with a tight-fitting lid in a cool, dark area for up to 3 months. These jars make attractive, inexpensive, and healing gifts!

Beautiful Bath

This bath of happiness is sure to invoke good memories and help bring all parts of your being into harmony. The all-natural benefits included in this blend are antidepressant, sedative, tonic, and restorative properties, to name a few. Baths can be so calming and restorative to someone suffering from bipolar illness, but adding these essential oils can just bring it to another level.

Yield: 1 application

RECIPE

5 drops melissa oil

5 drops frankincense oil

5 drops clary sage oil

1 tablespoon carrier oil

1 tablespoon milk (optional for adults, recommended for children)

As you begin to fill the tub with water, pour the chosen essential oils and carrier oil into the running water. Run a warm, not hot, bath. Water that is too hot will cause the essential oils to dissipate. You may add 1 tablespoon of milk to the water; this ensures that the essential oils will not stick to your skin, but will mix with the water. You

may soak in the water as long as you are comfortable. Dry your feet well once you get out of the water, as the oils will cause them to be slippery, increasing your chances of falling. Rinse the tub of any remaining oils.

Depression

There are many mood disorders, depression being one. There can be many reasons for depression. If a person has been diagnosed as clinically depressed, then they should be under a doctor's or therapist's supervision, as this condition can have dire consequences. Oftentimes a person feels lethargic or sad and does not seem to have an obvious reason for feeling this way. Essential oils have been used for thousands of years as a way of dispelling the feelings often associated with depression.

Essential Oils

Allspice, basil, bergamot, cedarwood, cinnamon, clary sage, cypress, frankincense, geranium, lemon, lime, marjoram, melaleuca, melissa, neroli, orange, patchouli, petit grain, rose, rosemary, sandalwood, vetiver, wild orange, and ylang-ylang

Smiling Again Massage

When you think that there is nothing you can do to regain your essential self, you can try some of these oils. Some of the therapeutic properties of this recipe include anti-depressant, hypotensive, and nervine agents.

Yield: 1 fluid ounce

RECIPE
3 drops vetiver oil
3 drops petitgrain oil
2 drops melissa oil
2 drops wild orange oil
2 drops lime oil
4 drops vitamin E oil
1 fluid ounce carrier oil

Pour the essential oils and the carrier oil into a small glass container, bowl, or jar. Swirl to mix the ingredients and use to massage lightly the area desired, such as temples, neck, chest, back, or soles of feet. Keep essential oil mixture away from open wounds, mucus membranes, genitals, eyes, and sensitive areas. Repeat application as needed. Store unused portion in a glass jar or container with a tight-fitting lid in a cool, dark area for up to 3 months.

Inhale My Blues Away

Do you need to lift your mood? Take a whiff of this aroma and you will feel great in no time. These essential oils work directly with the feel-good part of your brain and soul. The properties that induce these good feelings include antidepressant, aphrodisiac, tonic, and restorative components. This easy-to-use blend is one that I keep handy in a vial for quick use, and before you know it, I am feeling energized and happy.

Yield: 1 application

RECIPE
1 drop orange oil

or

1 drop lime oil

Choose your essential oil and apply to the palm of your hand, an oil inhaler, or a tissue. Bring the essential oils close to your nostrils and inhale the aroma deeply. You can cover one nostril at a time with your thumb and, if you prefer, alternate nostrils. This process sends the properties straight to your brain and the effects are immediate. You can complete this process 3–4 times daily.

Depression Diffuser

Unless you have been in the dark hole of depression yourself, it is so hard to understand how a person can't just "snap out of it." Using these essential oils will help with the therapeutic properties of antidepressant, tonic, and stimulating elements.

Yield: 1 application

RECIPE

2 drops jasmine oil

2 drops neroli oil

1 drop cinnamon oil

1 drop tea tree (melaleuca) oil

1 drop cedarwood oil

Water

Follow your directions for using essential oils in your particular brand of diffuser. Ensure that your diffuser does not use heat but runs by vibration, sound waves, or another cold-steam type of process. Choose the essential oils needed for your condition, then add water and oils to the diffuser. Run your diffuser as needed to permeate the air with therapeutic properties and achieve the results you desire.

Mellow Soak Bath Blend

Talk about mellow! This bath will get rid of the negativity and bring some positive influences into your life, your spirit, and your heart. These essential oils are known to bring peace and happiness to those who use them. The elements that boost your serotonin levels include antidepressant, restorative, and tonic-instilling agents.

Yield: 1 application

RECIPE

6 drops lavender oil

3 drops vetiver oil

2 drops orange oil

2 drops bergamot oil

1 tablespoon carrier oil

1 tablespoon milk (optional for adults, recommended for children)

As you begin to fill the tub with water, pour the chosen essential oils and carrier oil into the running water. Run a warm, not hot, bath. Water that is too hot will cause the essential oils to dissipate. You may add 1 tablespoon of milk to the water; this ensures that the essential oils will not stick to your skin, but will mix with the water. You

may soak in the water as long as you are comfortable. Dry your feet well once you get out of the water, as the oils will cause them to be slippery, increasing your chances of falling. Rinse the tub of any remaining oils.

Happy Bath Salts

These essential oils are perfect for rejuvenating and livening up the soul, spirit, and mind. They include antidepressant, tonic, and restorative properties. I adore this blend of oils and the wonderful aroma and positive energy they bring to me. They also instill some energy into my overly fatigued mind.

Yield: 3 cups

RECIPE

5 drops neroli oil

5 drops tea tree (melaleuca) oil

5 drops vetiver oil

5 drops jasmine oil

3 cups salts

5 drops vitamin E oil

2 tablespoons carrier oil

1 tablespoon milk (optional for adults, recommended for children)

Use any type of salt you prefer: pink Himalayan salt, sea salt, Epsom salts, etc. In a small container, add the essential oils to the desired type of salt. Stir until well blended. Screw lid onto container tightly. Leave mixture in a dark area for 24 hours and then stir mixture again. Run the bathwater. Once the tub is full of water, you can add the milk, and then add ½ cup of the bath salt mixture to bathwater as you get into the tub. You may stay in the tub as long as the temperature is comfortable. Dry your feet well when you get out of the bath, as the oils are slippery and can cause you to fall. Store remainder in a glass jar or container with a tight-fitting lid in a cool, dark area for up to 3 months. These jars make attractive, inexpensive, and healing gifts!

Detox

When one is ridding the body of substances that are harmful to one's well-being, or simply ridding the body of an accumulation of toxins, this is known as detoxing. Detox can often be used just to get the body refreshed and invigorated after a time of eating unhealthy food. Detox can also assist a person who wants to stop drinking alcohol, partaking in drugs, or smoking cigarettes. Essential oils can be beneficial in numerous facets of the detox process, from calming a person down during the withdrawal phase to distributing essential therapeutic properties throughout the body.

Essential Oils

Angelica, coriander, fennel, garlic, honeysuckle, juniper, lemon, peppermint, rose, and wild birch

Good Rub

Replace your bad habits with good ones. Apply a mixture of these essential oils each day to help you heal, have a great outlook, remain calm, and soothe the soul—as well as eliminate those nausea and stomach issues. The healing oils at work here contain depurative, digestive, stimulant, calming and stomachic therapeutic properties.

Yield: ½ ounce

RECIPE
3 drops coriander oil
3 drops grapefruit oil
1 drop fennel oil
2 drops juniper oil
3 drops vitamin E oil
½ ounce carrier oil

Pour the essential oils, carrier oil, and any remaining ingredients into a small glass container, bowl, or jar. Swirl or whisk to mix the ingredients and apply lightly to the area desired, such as pressure points, neck, soles of feet, temples, or chest. Keep essential oil mixture away from open wounds, mucus membranes, genitals, eyes, and sensitive areas. Repeat application as needed, usually 2–3 times daily. You may cover area with linen or cloth to protect clothing and furniture. Store unused portion in a glass jar or container with a tight-fitting lid in a cool, dark area for up to 3 months.

Detoxifying Air Cleanse

Run this diffuser to better your chances of making it through another day improving your lifestyle, mind, and health. These essential oils are reputed to keep you calm and focused on improving your life goals. Some of the calming and healing benefits in this recipe include aphrodisiac, stimulant, and nervine therapeutic properties.

Yield: 1 application

RECIPE
5 drops angelica oil
5 drops grapefruit oil
3 drops juniper oil
Water

Follow your directions for using essential oils in your particular brand of diffuser. Ensure that your diffuser does not use heat but runs by vibration, sound waves, or another cold-steam type of process. Choose the essential oils needed for your condition, then add water and oils to the diffuser. Run your diffuser as needed to permeate the air with therapeutic properties and achieve the results you desire.

Detox Bath Salts

The steam from the bath combined with these healing essential oils will help you to sweat out the toxins and get over that yucky pre-detox feeling and bring you closer to your perfect self. Just a few of the healing elements of this great blend include detoxifying, circulatory stimulant, depurative, diuretic, antitoxic, and tonic agents.

Yield: 3 cups

RECIPE
5 drops juniper oil
5 drops coriander oil

1 drop fennel oil

5 drops honeysuckle oil

2 tablespoons carrier oil

5 drops vitamin E oil

3 cups salts

1 tablespoon milk (optional for adults, recommended for children)

Use any type of salt you prefer: pink Himalayan salt, sea salt, Epsom salts, etc. In a small container, add the essential oils to the desired type of salt. Stir until well blended. Screw lid onto container tightly. Leave mixture in a dark area for 24 hours and then stir mixture again. Run the bathwater. Once the tub is full of water, you can add the milk, and then add ½ cup of the bath salt mixture to bathwater as you get into the tub. You may stay in the tub as long as the temperature is comfortable. Dry your feet well when you get out of the bath, as the oils are slippery and can cause you to fall. Store remainder in a glass jar or container with a tight-fitting lid in a cool, dark area for up to 3 months. These jars make attractive, inexpensive, and healing gifts!

Purifying Massage

These essential oils are reported to help rid the body of toxins and get you back to that pure, healthy state you desire with their antitoxic, circulatory stimulant, diuretic, and depurative properties.

Yield: 2 tablespoons

RECIPE

4 drops juniper oil

5 drops honeysuckle oil

1 drop peppermint oil

3 drops vitamin E oil

2 tablespoons carrier oil

Pour the essential oils and the carrier oil into a small glass container, bowl, or jar. Swirl to mix the ingredients and use to massage lightly the area desired, such as temples, neck, chest, back, or soles of feet. Keep essential oil mixture away from open wounds, mucus membranes, genitals, eyes, and sensitive areas. Repeat application as needed. Store unused portion in a glass jar or container with a tight-fitting lid in a cool, dark area for up to 3 months.

Fatigue

When a person is tired and does not feel like participating in daily activities but just wants to sleep, they may be just fatigued all the way to the soul. Fatigue is the feelings in the body letting a person know that they need sleep. Fatigue can also be an early signal that illness resides in the body. If fatigue is ongoing, a trip to your doctor for a clinical diagnosis may be in order. Essential oils can assist a person with calming the mind and relaxing enough to sleep, or to energize and renew the body for continuing with their responsibilities of life, the tasks at hand, and the joy of living.

Essential Oils

Angelica, basil, bergamot, black pepper, cinnamon, clove, cypress, eucalyptus, fir, ginger, grapefruit, lemon, lemongrass, patchouli, peppermint, pine, rosemary, sage, vetiver, and white fir

Wake Me Up Sugar Scrub

This recipe has the essential oils known for dispelling fatigue and giving the user a sense of ability to carry on and accomplish anything. These therapeutic properties work well together to bring focus, energy, and a bright attitude and to give you an overall feeling of power.

Yield: 8 ounces

RECIPE
8 ounces sugar (white or turbinado)
1 fluid ounce coconut oil
1 fluid ounce vegetable glycerin
1 fluid ounce liquid castile soap
½ teaspoon vitamin E oil
10 drops angelica oil

10 drops bergamot oil

10 drops grapefruit oil

10 drops lemongrass oil

10 drops patchouli oil

Combine ingredients without mashing too much. Spread paste onto skin or area desired and rub in lightly. Do not apply to genitals, eyes, sensitive areas, or mucus membranes. Sugar scrub should never be applied to the face. Let set for 1 minute, and then gently rise off. Keep in a glass jar with a tight-fitting lid in a cool, dark area for up to 1 month.

Power Up Bath

The benefits you will receive from this bath are open-mindedness, energy, and a positive outlook for the day ahead. These selected essential oils are full of energizing and stimulating properties to keep you alert throughout the day.

Yield: 1 application

RECIPE

3 drops angelica oil

3 drops grapefruit oil

3 drops citrus oil

2 drops cypress oil

1 drop lemongrass oil

1 tablespoon carrier oil

1 tablespoon milk (optional for adults, recommended for children)

As you begin to fill the tub with water, pour the chosen essential oils and carrier oil into the running water. Run a warm, not hot, bath. Water that is too hot will cause the essential oils to dissipate. You may add 1 tablespoon of milk to the water; this ensures that the essential oils will not stick to your skin, but will mix with the water. You may soak in the water as long as you are comfortable. Dry your feet well once you get out of the water, as the oils will cause them to be slippery, increasing your chances of falling. Rinse the tub of any remaining oils.

Energy Lip Balm

Use these energy-enhancing oils in a hurry with a quick swipe of your new favorite lip balm. These therapeutic properties will quickly be absorbed into your skin and the aromas will give energizing effects to your brain.

Yield: 1 tablespoon

RECIPE

3 teaspoons grape seed oil

½ teaspoon beeswax pellets

4 drops vitamin E oil

3 drops peppermint oil

3 drops pink grapefruit oil

Melt the beeswax and the carrier oil in a glass bowl in the microwave until most of the beeswax is melted. You can also use a pan on the stovetop on low. Cool slightly. Add the vitamin E and the essential oils and stir or whisk quickly. With a spoon, drip a drop of the mixture onto the counter and Let set for 1 minute. Pull your finger through the drop and check for consistency. If mixture is too thin, add more beeswax; if it is too thick, add more oil. Once desired consistency is acquired, immediately pour into small balm container (glass or metal) with a lid. After mixture cools, cover and store in a cool, dark area for up to 6 months.

Pick Me Up Footbath

Does anything feel better than a nice, peaceful footbath? Yes, a footbath with energizing essential oils in it! The essential oils will be transported through your feet and carried throughout your entire body to give you that huge burst of energy and get rid of every ounce of fatigue in your body. I love a good foot soak, and I especially love one that relaxes me for a while then gives me the desire to get up and do something.

Yield: 1 application

RECIPE

8 drops lemon oil

2 drops eucalyptus oil

2 drops peppermint oil

1 drop cinnamon oil

1 tablespoon carrier oil

1 tablespoon milk (optional for adults, recommended for children)

Combine all ingredients into a container large enough to comfortably rest your feet. Fill the container at least halfway with water that is not too hot, but as hot as you can comfortably stand it. Gently submerge your feet in the water and sit back and *relax*. Leave your feet in the footbath until the water is cool or uncomfortable, about 15 minutes. Dry feet and feel the energized peace you receive from this luxurious spa treatment. Discard water.

Energizing Bath Salts

I am a sucker for bath salts. This one is so energizing, exfoliating, and full of wonderful aromas along with healing and energy-boosting benefits. These amazing essential oils contain astringent, stimulant, and tonic therapeutic properties.

Yield: 3 cups

RECIPE

7 drops grapefruit oil

7 drops ginger oil

7 drops angelica oil

2 tablespoons carrier oil

5 drops vitamin E oil

3 cups salts

1 tablespoon milk (optional for adults, recommended for children)

Use any type of salt you prefer: pink Himalayan salt, sea salt, Epsom salts, etc. In a small container, add the essential oils to the desired type of salt. Stir until well blended. Screw lid onto container tightly. Leave mixture in a dark area for 24 hours and then stir mixture again. Run the bathwater. Once the tub is full of water, you can add the milk, and then add ½ cup of the bath salt mixture to bathwater as you get into the tub. You may stay in the tub as long as the temperature is comfortable. Dry your feet well when you get out of the bath, as the oils are slippery and can cause you

to fall. Store remainder in a glass jar or container with a tight-fitting lid in a cool, dark area for up to 3 months. These jars make attractive, inexpensive, and healing gifts!

Relaxing Spray

Oftentimes fatigue keeps us from sleeping because our worries and thoughts race through our minds. We are so tired that we can't keep our eyes open, but sleep remains elusive. This spray at bedtime can help you to relax, unwind, and fall gracefully into a peaceful, happy slumber.

Yield: 2 fluid ounces

RECIPE
10 drops angelica oil
10 drops vetiver oil
2 fluid ounces water
1 tablespoon witch hazel
3 drops vitamin E oil

Add all ingredients to a dark-colored spray bottle. Check for material steadfastness before spraying on fabric. Shake the bottle and spray onto area desired, such as body, hair, home, car, or office. Do not spray into or on open wounds, genitals, eyes, or mucus membranes. Store in a cool, dark area for up to 3 months. Shake well before each use to combine the ingredients.

Forgetfulness

Forgetting things can happen due to numerous factors such as aging, illness, fatigue, and a host of other deciding variables. There are several things that a person can do to increase memory skills: puzzles, reading, learning a new language, and repeating phrases, to name a few. Essential oils are reputed to assist with memory enhancement, and it's never too late to start remembering.

Essential Oils

Basil, citrus, clary sage, cypress, frankincense, lavender, lemon, lemongrass, marjoram, melissa, orange, patchouli, peppermint, rosemary, and vetiver

Back in Time Powder

Put some of this powder between your sheets and let it work all night to instill the mysteries of memories long in the past into your brain. These essential oils are known to bring back long-forgotten memories and increase short-term memory skills as well.

Yield: ¼ cup

RECIPE

3 drops basil oil

7 drops vetiver oil

3 drops melissa oil

4 drops vitamin E oil

¼ cup cornstarch

Place the ingredients into a mason jar, stirring well with a whisk. Carefully poke holes into the lid, use this as a shaker, and shake the ingredients into pillowcases or under sheet areas as needed. You can get a piece of plastic wrap and place it over the jar and under the lid to keep powder from spilling out when not in use. Store in a glass jar or container with a tight-fitting lid in a cool, dark, and dry area for up to 3 months.

Remember Rub

This rub has been said to increase memory skills and help improve short-term memory loss. Use these essential oils repeatedly to keep improving your memory as time goes on.

Yield: 1 application

RECIPE

3 drops peppermint oil

2 drops frankincense oil

> 1 drop melissa oil
>
> 1 teaspoon carrier oil
>
> 3 drops vitamin E oil

Pour the essential oils, carrier oil, and any remaining ingredients into a small glass container, bowl, or jar. Swirl or whisk to mix the ingredients and apply lightly to the area desired, such as pressure points, neck, soles of feet, temples, or chest. Keep essential oil mixture away from open wounds, mucus membranes, genitals, eyes, and sensitive areas. Repeat application as needed, usually 2–3 times daily. You may cover area with linen or cloth to protect clothing and furniture. Store unused portion in a glass jar or container with a tight-fitting lid in a cool, dark area for up to 3 months.

Memory Diffuser

This recipe is full of essential oils that are said to jog the memory when you are regularly trying to remember the recent past as if it's on the tip of your tongue but you can never remember. It has often been stated that the best memory enabler is smell. Some of the aromas here will spark those memory receptors in the brain, bring peaceful memories, and improve memory lapses in all who inhale this delightful aroma.

Yield: 1 application

RECIPE

> 3 drops peppermint oil
>
> 2 drops vetiver oil
>
> 2 drops melissa oil
>
> Water

Follow your directions for using essential oils in your particular brand of diffuser. Ensure that your diffuser does not use heat but runs by vibration, sound waves, or another cold-steam type of process. Choose the essential oils needed for your condition, then add water and oils to the diffuser. Run your diffuser as needed to permeate the air with therapeutic properties and achieve the results you desire.

Focusing Remedy

These essential oils should help you to focus and to remember those answers you need for whatever project, whether it be an interview, a task, or a test. These essential oils are known for their memory-retaining properties. Try this rub in the morning before school and watch your memory and test-taking skills increase. Good luck!

Yield: 1 application

RECIPE
1 drop sandalwood oil
1 drop frankincense oil
1 drop patchouli oil
1 drop lime oil
1 teaspoon carrier oil

Pour the essential oils and the carrier oil into a small glass container, bowl, or jar. Swirl to mix the ingredients and use to massage lightly the area desired, such as temples, neck, chest, back, or soles of feet. Keep essential oil mixture away from open wounds, mucus membranes, genitals, eyes, and sensitive areas. Repeat application as needed. Store unused portion in a glass jar or container with a tight-fitting lid in a cool, dark area for up to 3 months.

Memory Inhale

A quick memory instiller that only takes a second but often has long-lasting dramatic results. Carry these essential oils with you and smell before that presentation or speaking engagement.

Yield: 1 application

RECIPE
1 drop peppermint oil
or
1 drop frankincense oil

Choose your essential oil and apply to the palm of your hand, an oil inhaler, or a tissue. Bring the essential oils close to your nostrils and inhale the aroma deeply. You can cover one nostril at a time with your thumb and, if you prefer, alternate nostrils. This process sends the properties straight to your brain and the effects are immediate. You can complete this procedure 3–4 times daily.

Memory-Boosting Rub

The feet are thought to be one of the best areas on the body to put essential oils. The feet quickly absorb the healing properties in the oils and take the therapeutic properties to every cell in the body, and to the parts of the body where they are most needed—in this case, the memory portion of the brain. These oils have long been used to stimulate your brain and help you to remember things better day to day.

Yield: 1–2 applications

RECIPE
3 drops vetiver oil
3 drops peppermint oil
1 tablespoon carrier oil

Pour the essential oils, carrier oil, and any remaining ingredients into a small glass container, bowl, or jar. Swirl or whisk to mix the ingredients and apply lightly to the area desired, such as pressure points, neck, soles of feet, temples, or chest. Keep essential oil mixture away from open wounds, mucus membranes, genitals, eyes, and sensitive areas. Repeat application as needed, usually 2–3 times daily. You may cover area with linen or cloth to protect clothing and furniture. Store unused portion in a glass jar or container with a tight-fitting lid in a cool, dark area for up to 3 months.

Memory Bath Salts

Soak in a tub with these oils and remember pleasant thoughts and events from the past. These essential oils increase memory for hours in your body and will have long-lasting effects throughout the night, giving you dreams that are full of loved ones and memories from the past.

Yield: 3 cups

RECIPE

5 drops orange oil

5 drops lavender oil

5 drops clary sage oil

5 drops vetiver oil

2 tablespoons carrier oil

5 drops vitamin E oil

3 cups salts

1 tablespoon milk (optional for adults, recommended for children)

Use any type of salt you prefer: pink Himalayan salt, sea salt, Epsom salts, etc. In a small container, add the essential oils to the desired type of salt. Stir until well blended. Screw lid onto container tightly. Leave mixture in a dark area for 24 hours and then stir mixture again. Run the bathwater. Once the tub is full of water, you can add the milk, and then add ½ cup of the bath salt mixture to bathwater as you get into the tub. You may stay in the tub as long as the temperature is comfortable. Dry your feet well when you get out of the bath, as the oils are slippery and can cause you to fall. Store remainder in a glass jar or container with a tight-fitting lid in a cool, dark area for up to 3 months. These jars make attractive, inexpensive, and healing gifts!

Grief

Grief is the sadness, despair, and heartache that usually accompanies the death of a close loved one, but grief can also be experienced due to life events such as divorce, moving, or ending a friendship or career. Persons suffering from grief can often present to the outward world that they are okay, but inside they feel as if they themselves are dying, or wish that they were. The properties in these essential oils can help a person to learn again to experience joy and happiness and, most importantly, an inward calmness, peace, and serenity.

Essential Oils

Basil, cassia, citrus, cypress, frankincense, geranium, grapefruit, lemon, lime, rose, sandalwood, vetiver, and ylang-ylang

Archer's Grief Powder

Everyone must grieve for the loss in their life in order to have complete healing. These essential oils are reported to help you get through the grief process more easily. These antidepressant, sedative, and tranquilizing properties will work together to bring much-needed deep sleep in times of grief.

Yield: ¼ cup

RECIPE

3 drops vetiver oil

3 drops geranium oil

3 drops citrus oil

6 drops frankincense oil

4 drops vitamin E oil

¼ cup cornstarch

Place the ingredients into a mason jar, stirring well with a whisk. Carefully poke holes into the lid, use this as a shaker, and shake the ingredients into pillowcases or under sheet areas as needed. You can get a piece of plastic wrap and place it over the jar and under the lid to keep powder from spilling out when not in use. Store in a glass jar or container with a tight-fitting lid in a cool, dark, and dry area for up to 3 months.

Reassuring Bath Salts

This bath will help you to feel better and like you might want to truly live life again. Give it a try the next time you feel you just can't go on another day. These essential oils will give you the strength through their antidepressant and tonic-inducing therapeutic properties.

Yield: 3 cups

RECIPE

5 drops orange oil

5 drops frankincense oil

5 drops vetiver oil

2 tablespoons carrier oil

5 drops vitamin E oil

3 cups salts

1 tablespoon milk (optional for adults, recommended for children)

Use any type of salt you prefer: pink Himalayan salt, sea salt, Epsom salts, etc. In a small container, add the essential oils to the desired type of salt. Stir until well blended. Screw lid onto container tightly. Leave mixture in a dark area for 24 hours and then stir mixture again. Run the bathwater. Once the tub is full of water, you can add the milk, and then add ½ cup of the bath salt mixture to bathwater as you get into the tub. You may stay in the tub as long as the temperature is comfortable. Dry your feet well when you get out of the bath, as the oils are slippery and can cause you to fall. Store remainder in a glass jar or container with a tight-fitting lid in a cool, dark area for up to 3 months. These jars can also make attractive, inexpensive, and healing gifts!

Sadness Dispelling Diffuser

This diffuser recipe has the essential oils needed to bring positive energy in and to get all of the negative energy out. Life force–enhancing antidepressant, aphrodisiacal, and euphoric properties work to give you the boost you need to live life to its fullest.

Yield: 1 application

RECIPE

4 drops vetiver oil

3 drops rose oil

3 drops ylang-ylang oil

Water

Follow your directions for using essential oils in your particular brand of diffuser. Ensure that your diffuser does not use heat but runs by vibration, sound waves, or an-

other cold-steam type of process. Choose the essential oils needed for your condition, then add water and oils to the diffuser. Run your diffuser as needed to permeate the air with therapeutic properties and achieve the results you desire.

Inhale Some Happiness

This recipe is an instant grief dispeller to help you face the future with the best of intentions. The essential oils in this recipe are reputed to bring happiness and peace with their antidepressant, euphoric, and mood-boosting properties.

Yield: 1 application

RECIPE
1 drop frankincense oil

or

1 drop vetiver oil

or

1 drop lemon oil

Choose your essential oil and apply to the palm of your hand, an oil inhaler, or a tissue. Bring the essential oils close to your nostrils and inhale the aroma deeply. You can cover one nostril at a time with your thumb and, if you prefer, alternate nostrils. This process sends the properties straight to your brain and the effects are immediate. You can complete this process 3–4 times daily.

Bathing in Happiness

This is the perfect bath to take when you are feeling down and full of grief. The essential oils will help you to get through that grieving process. This recipe has aphrodisiac, harmonizing, and tonic therapeutic properties to bring happiness to your mind, body, soul, and spirit.

Yield: 1 application

RECIPE
4 drops sandalwood oil
3 drops sweet orange oil

2 drops cypress oil

1 tablespoon carrier oil

1 tablespoon milk (optional for adults, recommended for children)

As you begin to fill the tub with water, pour the chosen essential oils and carrier oil into the running water. Run a warm, not hot, bath. Water that is too hot will cause the essential oils to dissipate. You may add 1 tablespoon of milk to the water; this ensures that the essential oils will not stick to your skin, but will mix with the water. You may soak in the water as long as you are comfortable. Dry your feet well once you get out of the water, as the oils will cause them to be slippery, increasing your chances of falling. Rinse the tub of any remaining oils.

Coming to Terms Rub

Learning to advance through the stages of grief is a very painful process emotionally and spiritually. These oils are reported to assist you with navigating these stages and ease your mind and soul. These oils have tonic, aphrodisiac, and natural elevating/harmonizing properties.

Yield: 2 fluid ounces

RECIPE

4 drops cypress oil

5 drops frankincense oil

5 drops sandalwood oil

8 drops vetiver oil

3 drops vitamin E oil

2 fluid ounces carrier oil

Pour the essential oils, carrier oil, and any remaining ingredients into a small glass container, bowl, or jar. Swirl or whisk to mix the ingredients and apply lightly to the area desired, such as pressure points, neck, soles of feet, temples, or chest. Keep essential oil mixture away from open wounds, mucus membranes, genitals, eyes, and sensitive areas. Repeat application as needed, usually 2–3 times daily. You may cover area with linen or cloth to protect clothing and furniture. Store unused portion in a glass jar or container with a tight-fitting lid in a cool, dark area for up to 3 months.

Hangover

The physical characteristics a person experiences after consuming a certain amount of alcohol is widely known as a hangover. Usually, the next day the person is disoriented and nauseous, and has digestive issues, a headache, and other uncomfortable side effects. Essential oils can help you overcome many of the ill effects of alcohol.

Essential Oils

Rosemary, rose, juniper, lemon, lavender, grapefruit, ginger, and sandalwood

Hangover Bath Salts

This bath will quiet your disparaging questions of "What the heck did I do?" and bring you back to a more pleasant state of mind. The essential oils in this recipe were distilled from plants used for centuries to end the hangover blues. They contain antidepressant, antirheumatic, antitoxic, and antispasmodic elements to ease you mentally and physically.

Yield: 3 cups

RECIPE

7 drops rose oil

7 drops juniper oil

7 drops lavender oil

5 drops vitamin E oil

2 tablespoons carrier oil

3 cups salts

1 tablespoon milk (optional)

Use any type of salt you prefer: pink Himalayan salt, sea salt, Epsom salts, etc. In a small container, add the essential oils to the desired type of salt. Stir until well blended. Screw lid onto container tightly. Leave mixture in a dark area for 24 hours and then stir mixture again. Run the bathwater. Once the tub is full of water, you can add the milk, and then add ½ cup of the bath salt mixture to bathwater as you get into the tub. You may stay in the tub as long as the temperature is comfortable. Dry your feet well when you get out of the bath, as the oils are slippery and can cause you to fall. Store remainder in a glass jar or container with a tight-fitting lid in a cool, dark area for up to 3 months. These jars make attractive, inexpensive, and healing gifts!

Sober Air

This recipe is one used for a long time in the United States. Aromas play an important role in recovering from a hangover. The next time you have a little too much fun, try this blend and see how much better you feel on that miserable day after.

Yield: 1 application

RECIPE
5 drops grapefruit oil
4 drops sandalwood oil
Water

Follow your directions for using essential oils in your particular brand of diffuser. Ensure that your diffuser does not use heat but runs by vibration, sound waves, or another cold-steam type of process. Choose the essential oils needed for your condition, then add water and oils to the diffuser. Run your diffuser as needed to permeate the air with therapeutic properties and achieve the results you desire.

Nausea No More

This is a little trick I use when I am feeling nauseated and have an important task to complete. It's easy and quick and works wonders for that headache, nausea, and fatigue.

Yield: 1 application

RECIPE
1 drop lemon oil
or
1 drop ginger oil

Choose your essential oil and apply to the palm of your hand, an oil inhaler, or a tissue. Bring the essential oils close to your nostrils and inhale the aroma deeply. You can cover one nostril at a time with your thumb and, if you prefer, alternate nostrils. This process sends the properties straight to your brain and the effects are immediate. You can complete this procedure 3–4 times daily.

Hopelessness

Oftentimes we feel hopeless about a situation, an illness, a loved one's predicament, or our lives in general. Immersing ourselves in essential oils have been known to impart a feeling of hope and to help us to reflect on how we can help ourselves or others in a bleak situation. These essential oils listed below have been reported throughout history to not only help us to renew our hope, but to also help make our hopes and dreams a reality.

Essential Oils

Bergamot, frankincense, grapefruit, lavender, lemon, lime, melissa, peppermint, Roman chamomile, rosemary, and ylang-ylang

Hope Upon Hope Linen Powder

Sleep on this powder and wake in the morning with a new outlook and a more positive approach to life. This recipe contains essential oils reputed widely for their hopeful and uniquely positive benefits.

Yield: ¼ cup

RECIPE
3 drops grapefruit oil
3 drops lavender oil
3 drops chamomile oil
4 drops vitamin E oil
¼ cup cornstarch

Place the ingredients into a mason jar, stirring well with a whisk. Carefully poke holes into the lid, use this as a shaker, and shake the ingredients into pillowcases or under

sheet areas as needed. You can get a piece of plastic wrap and place it over the jar and under the lid to keep powder from spilling out when not in use. Store in a glass jar or container with a tight-fitting lid in a cool, dark, and dry area for up to 3 months.

Hopeful Bath Salts

Do you have a secret hope for yourself or a loved one's future? Finding hope is sometimes all we have to cling to. Soak yourself in these essential oils to renew hope, energize, and give yourself a fighting chance at life and all of its intricacies.

Yield: 3 cups

RECIPE
7 drops Roman chamomile oil
7 drops ylang-ylang oil
7 drops melissa oil
2 tablespoons carrier oil
4 drops vitamin E oil
3 cups salts
1 tablespoon milk (optional for adults, recommended for children)

Use any type of salt you prefer: pink Himalayan salt, sea salt, Epsom salts, etc. In a small container, add the essential oils to the desired type of salt. Stir until well blended. Screw lid onto container tightly. Leave mixture in a dark area for 24 hours and then stir mixture again. Run the bathwater. Once the tub is full of water, you can add the milk, and then add ½ cup of the bath salt mixture to bathwater as you get into the tub. You may stay in the tub as long as the temperature is comfortable. Dry your feet well when you get out of the bath, as the oils are slippery and can cause you to fall. Store remainder in a glass jar or container with a tight-fitting lid in a cool, dark area for up to 3 months. These jars make attractive, inexpensive, and healing gifts!

Renewing Hope Massage

When you feel you are at the last straw and have lost all hope, this massage will give you the strength to renew your hope and determination to get the deed done. This recipe has the essential oils that people have used to restore their hope for the future for ages.

Yield: 2 fluid ounces

RECIPE
4 drops bergamot oil
3 drops grapefruit oil
3 drops lemon oil
1 drop melissa oil
3 drops vitamin E oil
2 fluid ounces carrier oil

Pour the essential oils and the carrier oil into a small glass container, bowl, or jar. Swirl to mix the ingredients and use to massage lightly the area desired, such as temples, neck, chest, back, or soles of feet. Keep essential oil mixture away from open wounds, mucus membranes, genitals, eyes, and sensitive areas. Repeat application as needed. Store unused portion in a glass jar or container with a tight-fitting lid in a cool, dark area for up to 3 months.

Hope is in the Air

To get the crowd on board with you and to motivate others, this is the perfect blend of essential oils to get them going. These essential oils are motivating and inspiring and help to renew that sense of hope and wonder.

Yield: 1 application

RECIPE
2 drops frankincense oil
2 drops lavender oil
2 drops Roman chamomile oil
Water

Follow your directions for using essential oils in your particular brand of diffuser. Ensure that your diffuser does not use heat but runs by vibration, sound waves, or another cold-steam type of process. Choose the essential oils needed for your condition, then add water and oils to the diffuser. Run your diffuser as needed to permeate the air with therapeutic properties and achieve the results you desire.

Keep the Faith Rub

Some call these essential oils lucky, some call them invigorating, but whatever you use them for, they will renew your hope and faith in humankind and yourself.

Yield: 1 fluid ounce

RECIPE

7 drops lime oil

4 drops peppermint oil

2 drops rosemary oil

3 drops vitamin E oil

1 fluid ounce carrier oil

Pour the essential oils, carrier oil, and any remaining ingredients into a small glass container, bowl, or jar. Swirl or whisk to mix the ingredients and apply lightly to the area desired, such as pressure points, neck, soles of feet, temples, or chest. Keep essential oil mixture away from open wounds, mucus membranes, genitals, eyes, and sensitive areas. Repeat application as needed, usually 2–3 times daily. You may cover area with linen or cloth to protect clothing and furniture. Store unused portion in a glass jar or container with a tight-fitting lid in a cool, dark area for up to 3 months.

Keeping Up the Spirit Bath

Bathe with these essential oils to renew your spirit, faith, and hope for others and yourself. Oftentimes we lose faith and hope in our beliefs, our love, our ideas or our friends. Relax in these essential oils and concentrate on renewing your hope. Sometimes hope is all we have.

Yield: 1 application

RECIPE

5 drops bergamot oil

4 drops frankincense oil

2 drops grapefruit oil

2 drops lavender oil

1 tablespoon carrier oil

1 tablespoon milk (optional for adults, recommended for children)

As you begin to fill the tub with water, pour the chosen essential oils and carrier oil into the running water. Run a warm, not hot, bath. Water that is too hot will cause the essential oils to dissipate. You may add 1 tablespoon of milk to the water; this ensures that the essential oils will not stick to your skin, but will mix with the water. You may soak in the water as long as you are comfortable. Dry your feet well once you get out of the water, as the oils will cause them to be slippery, increasing your chances of falling. Rinse the tub of any remaining oils.

Positively Hopeful Spray

This recipe works well to use in the home, office, or car to increase hope and positivity in all who come in contact with the aroma. These oils have been used for thousands of years to inspire, lift, and encourage the good in all people.

Yield: 2 fluid ounces

RECIPE

11 drops ylang-ylang oil

3 drops lemon oil

3 drops Roman chamomile oil

3 drops bergamot oil

1 tablespoon witch hazel

2 fluid ounces water

Add all ingredients to a dark-colored spray bottle. Check for material steadfastness before spraying on fabric. Shake the bottle and spray onto area desired, such as body, hair, home, car, or office. Do not spray into or on open wounds, genitals, eyes, or mucus membranes. Store in a cool, dark area for up to 3 months. Shake well before each use to combine the ingredients.

Breath of Hope Inhale

Carry a vial of these essential oils with you wherever you go so that you can use them at a moment's notice. These essential oils are known all over the world for their hope-inducing properties and benefits.

Yield: 1 application

RECIPE
1 drop lavender oil

or

1 drop of frankincense oil

or

1 drop of bergamot oil

Choose your essential oil and apply to the palm of your hand, an oil inhaler, or a tissue. Bring the essential oils close to your nostrils and inhale the aroma deeply. You can cover one nostril at a time with your thumb and, if you prefer, alternate nostrils. This process sends the properties straight to your brain and the effects are immediate. You can complete this procedure 3–4 times daily.

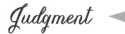

Judgment

Judging others is something that we don't want to be guilty of, but we often are. We are all judgmental to an extent. We learn to protect ourselves by judging if someone is who they project themselves to be. We do not want to be overly friendly with a pathological, lying drama queen, so we try to distance ourselves from people like that. Then again, people are judging us at the same time. Are we who we are presenting ourselves to be? I try not to judge others, but am extremely guilty of judging myself every day. These essential oils are used to help us learn to not judge others, help others to not judge us too harshly, and to be more lenient when judging ourselves.

Essential Oils

Bergamot, cajuput, cypress, elemi, frankincense, juniper, lavender, neroli, rose, rosewood, and wild orange

Scales of Justice Spray

This spray has the therapeutic properties to calm my anxiety about myself, and others. I have had great success using this on myself or on my surroundings when given the chance to use it. These oils will help us to be calmer, more relaxed, and open to others, and help others to be more open to us.

Yield: 2 fluid ounces

RECIPE

7 drops elemi oil

3 drops rosewood oil

3 drops frankincense oil

3 drops cypress oil

1 tablespoon witch hazel

2 fluid ounces water

Add all ingredients to a dark-colored spray bottle. Check for material steadfastness before spraying on fabric. Shake the bottle and spray onto area desired, such as body, hair, home, car, or office. Do not spray into or on open wounds, genitals, eyes, or mucus membranes. Store in a cool, dark area for up to 3 months. Shake well before each use to combine the ingredients.

Clear the Air

This diffuser recipe is one I often use to dispel any form of judgments that I believe may be going on in my own household. These oils impart wisdom- and patience-inducing properties.

Yield: 1 application

RECIPE

3 drops cajuput oil

3 drops bergamot oil

3 drops rose oil

Water

Follow your directions for using essential oils in your particular brand of diffuser. Ensure that your diffuser does not use heat but runs by vibration, sound waves, or another cold-steam type of process. Choose the essential oils needed for your condition, then add water and oils to the diffuser. Run your diffuser as needed to permeate the air with therapeutic properties and achieve the results you desire.

Judge Me Not

This is a quick little dab you can use when you are about to be confronted with someone who you know does not bring positive energy your way. Oftentimes we must deal with people who are very negative and talk badly about others. When I am at work or in public, I can't whip out my spray, but I can (and do) excuse myself for a moment and dab this on in a second. Frankincense brings a sense of peace, non-judgment, calm, and goodwill to me and to others.

Yield: 1 application

RECIPE
1 drop frankincense oil

Apply to the palm of your hand, an oil inhaler, or a tissue. Bring the essential oil close to your nostrils and inhale the aroma deeply. You can cover one nostril at a time with your thumb and, if you prefer, alternate nostrils. This process sends the properties straight to your brain and the effects are immediate. You can complete this procedure 3–4 times daily.

Melancholy

That sad, wistful, numbing emotion that sometimes overtakes us all. We can live in our heads with thoughts of "what if …" or "I wish I wouldn't have …", but the emotion of melancholy can sometimes lead to the more serious mood of depression. To help yourself or a loved one enjoy the emotions of gratitude, bliss, and joy, use one of these essential oils that have been used forever to bring comfort and happiness.

Essential Oils

Angelica, bergamot, basil, bay laurel, clary sage, helichrysum, jasmine, melissa, orange, Palo Santo, tangerine, and St. John's wort

Lift the Spirits Sugar Scrub

This recipe can take you from low spirits to high spirits and relieve that mood that has you down. These essential oils are well known for their mood-lifting therapeutic properties.

Yield: 8 ounces

RECIPE

8 ounces sugar (white or turbinado)

1 fluid ounce coconut oil

1 fluid ounce vegetable glycerin

1 fluid ounce liquid castile soap

½ teaspoon vitamin E oil

10 drops angelica oil

10 drops tangerine oil

10 drops St. John's wort oil

10 drops Palo Santo oil

10 drops bay laurel oil

Combine ingredients without mashing too much. Spread paste onto skin or area desired and rub in lightly. Do not apply to genitals, eyes, sensitive areas, or mucus membranes. Sugar scrub should never be applied to the face. Let set for 1 minute, and then gently rise off. Keep in a glass jar with a tight-fitting lid in a cool, dark area for up to 1 month.

Beautiful Life Bath and Shower Bombs

I like to make these bath and shower bombs when I am experiencing sadness due to personal issues. The essential oils in this blend relax a person and help to make their thoughts turn to more pleasant memories, dreams, and hopes.

Yield: 8–12 bombs

RECIPE

1 cup baking soda

½ cup citric acid

½ cup cornstarch

½ cup Epsom salts, fine grained

15 drops bay laurel oil

15 drops tangerine oil

5 drops melissa oil

½ teaspoon carrier oil

¾ teaspoon water

spray bottle (water)

In a large bowl, mix your dry ingredients together until fine with a whisk. In a tiny jar with a lid, add your wet ingredients and shake to mix. You may add a couple drops of food coloring to the wet jar. Extremely slowly, add the wet ingredients to the dry ingredients while whisking rapidly. If fizzing takes place, whisk until it is mixed. Once the ingredients are well mixed, it should be the texture of slightly damp sand. Add a spray or two of water if needed. Once the mixture is the consistency you like, form into balls; I just smash mine down into ice cube trays or muffin tins. You can use cute molds, but you must work rapidly as mixture will dry out quickly. Leave in open air, uncovered, in a room where they will not be disturbed for 12–24 hours. Once they are dry, you can place 1–2 bombs into your bath or directly into the spray of the shower and they will fizz and release their aromatic and healing properties. Store unused portion in an airtight container for up to 6 months.

Gentle Breeze Footbath

This luxurious footbath will calm the mind and bring peace to a troubled spirit. These oils have tranquilizing, sedative, and calming therapeutic properties to help relax an overactive mind.

Yield: 1 application

RECIPE
5 drops bergamot oil
5 drops St. John's wort oil
3 drops basil oil
1 quart water
1 tablespoon milk (optional for adults, recommended for children)

Combine the oils, milk and any other ingredients into a container large enough to comfortably rest your feet. Fill the container at least half way with water that is not too hot, but as hot as you can comfortably stand it. Gently submerge your feet in the water and sit back and Relax. Leave your feet in the footbath until the water is cool or uncomfortable, about 15 minutes. Dry feet and feel the energized peace you receive from this luxurious spa treatment. Discard water.

Nature's Wonders Hand Rub

One of the most pleasant, relaxing, and quick-working remedies in essential oils. This hand rub contains essential oils that will bring peace and happiness to a troubled soul.

Yield: 1–2 applications

RECIPE
3 drops angelica oil
3 drops melissa oil
2 drops bergamot oil
2 drops vitamin E oil (optional)
Enough warm water to fill bowl halfway

Combine the ingredients together into a small bowl. Dip one hand into the bowl until fingers are covered in the oils. Rub hands together for 5–15 minutes, rinse if desired, and repeat as often as needed. Ensure that the oils have been completely absorbed into your skin before touching furniture, clothing, etc., or oils may stain. I sometimes wear gloves throughout the night over the oils to ensure that the therapeutic properties are absorbed to their fullest all night long. Pour remainder into a jar with a tight-fitting lid, and store in a cool, dark area for up to 1 month.

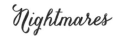

Nightmares

Oftentimes young children have nightmares that disrupt the sleep of the entire household. Nightmares can affect persons of any age and can be related to stress, overwork, and traumatic situations. Essential oils can help people to calm their brain patterns and sleep more easily with the sedative, tranquilizing, and calming therapeutic properties. Never use essential oils on a child under the age of four years without specific instruction from a certified aromatherapist.

Essential Oils

Basil, bergamot, chamomile, clary sage, frankincense, lavender, mandarin, and sandalwood

Sweet Dreams Bath

This is a recipe for good dreams and happy memories at night. Calming and soothing agents work together to reduce the stress related to nightmares. This blend includes antidepressant, sedative, and nervine properties.

Yield: 1 application

RECIPE
5 drops clary sage oil
5 drops mandarin oil
5 drops bergamot oil
1 tablespoon carrier oil
1 tablespoon milk (optional for adults, recommended for children)

As you begin to fill the tub with water, pour the chosen essential oils and carrier oil into the running water. Run a warm, not hot, bath. Water that is too hot will cause the essential oils to dissipate. You may add 1 tablespoon of milk to the water; this ensures that the essential oils will not stick to your skin, but will mix with the water. You

may soak in the water as long as you are comfortable. Dry your feet well once you get out of the water, as the oils will cause them to be slippery, increasing your chances of falling. Rinse the tub of any remaining oils.

Dusk to Dawn Air

Run this diffuser an hour ahead of bedtime to get the children in the mood for a happy, peaceful night's sleep with its antidepressant, sedative, analgesic, and warming properties.

Yield: 1 application

RECIPE
5 drops chamomile oil
3 drops bergamot oil
Water

Follow your directions for using essential oils in your particular brand of diffuser. Ensure that your diffuser does not use heat but runs by vibration, sound waves, or another cold-steam type of process. Choose the essential oils needed for your condition, then add water and oils to the diffuser. Run your diffuser as needed to permeate the air with therapeutic properties and achieve the results you desire.

Floating Cloud Inhaler

When someone wakes up in the middle of the night with night terrors, one smell of a drop of either of these essential oils can help to allay their fears and they can return to bed with no worries of terrors invading their sleep again. These oils contain antidepressant and sedative properties.

Yield: 1 application

RECIPE
1 drop sandalwood oil
or
1 drop lavender oil
or
1 drop clary sage oil

Choose your essential oil and apply to the palm of your hand, an oil inhaler, or a tissue. Bring the essential oils close to your nostrils and inhale the aroma deeply. You can cover one nostril at a time with your thumb and, if you prefer, alternate nostrils. This process sends the properties straight to your brain and the effects are immediate. You can complete this procedure in the middle of the night quickly and easily. Just have a bottle handy, but in a safe place, that you can grab easily the next time your child has night terrors.

Monster Zapper Spray

This spray is a great way to help children (over the age of four years) get back to sleep. They can take the power into their own hands when equipped with this monster zapping spray. The sleep-inducing (and monster inhibiting) properties include antidepressant, nervine, and sedative agents, which are great for adults too.

Yield: 2 fluid ounces

RECIPE
5 drops bergamot oil
5 drops frankincense oil
3 drops mandarin oil
3 drops clary sage oil
1 tablespoon witch hazel
2 fluid ounces water

Add all ingredients to a dark-colored spray bottle. Check for material steadfastness before spraying on fabric. Shake the bottle and spray onto area desired, such as body, hair, home, car, or office. Do not spray into or on open wounds, genitals, eyes, or mucus membranes. Store in a cool, dark area for up to 3 months. Shake well before each use to combine the ingredients.

Monster Bombs

Let your child throw this bath bomb in the tub and take control of their own bath time and bedtime rituals, as long as they are over the age of four years old. They don't know that the properties in these oils will help them to drift off into an easy, peaceful slumber. Adults can benefit the same way children can with these calming bath bombs.

Yield: 8–12 bombs

RECIPE

1 cup baking soda

½ cup citric acid

½ cup cornstarch

½ cup Epsom salts, fine grained

15 drops lavender oil

15 drops mandarin oil

½ teaspoon carrier oil

¾ teaspoon water

spray bottle (water)

In a large bowl, mix your dry ingredients together until fine with a whisk. In a tiny jar with a lid, add your wet ingredients and shake to mix. You may add a couple drops of food coloring to the wet jar. Extremely slowly, add the wet ingredients to the dry ingredients while whisking rapidly. If fizzing takes place, whisk until it is mixed. Once the ingredients are well mixed, it should be the texture of slightly damp sand. Add a spray or two of water if needed. Once the mixture is the consistency you like, form into balls; I just smash mine down into ice cube trays or muffin tins. You can use cute molds, but you must work rapidly as mixture will dry out quickly. Leave in open air, uncovered, in a room where they will not be disturbed for 12–24 hours. Once they are dry, you can place 1–2 bombs into your bath or directly into the spray of the shower and they will fizz and release their aromatic and healing properties. Store unused portion in an airtight container for up to 6 months.

OCD (Obsessive-Compulsive Disorder)

When a person has the same thoughts of worry over and over, this is a type of OCD. There are various branches of OCD and the thought patterns that accompany OCD are very hard to break. Locking and unlocking doors repeatedly, excessively cleaning and organizing, washing hands repeatedly, and counting and repeating words are all forms of OCD. New medications offer hope and wellness to many who have suffered from chronic OCD and they are available today. Therapy has also proven to be very useful in treating OCD patients. Essential oils can be used to bring calmness to a situation and decrease the behaviors where someone suffering from OCD could have a troubling time.

Essential Oils

Clary sage, cypress, frankincense, geranium, lavender, patchouli, vetiver, and ylang-ylang

Train of Thought Massage

These essential oils will help you to multitask and not be so obsessed over the invading matters that are constantly at the forefront of your thoughts. This blend contains antidepressant, nervine, and sedative properties.

Yield: 2 fluid ounces

RECIPE
8 drops frankincense oil
4 drops cypress oil
4 drops ylang-ylang oil
4 drops vitamin E oil
2 fluid ounces carrier oil

Pour the essential oils and the carrier oil into a small glass container, bowl, or jar. Swirl to mix the ingredients and use to massage lightly the area desired, such as temples, neck, chest, back, or soles of feet. Keep essential oil mixture away from open wounds, mucus membranes, genitals, eyes, and sensitive areas. Repeat application as needed. Store unused portion in a glass jar or container with a tight-fitting lid in a cool, dark area for up to 3 months.

Peaceful Powder

This linen powder recipe contains the essential oils that calm the brain and help a person to think more positive thoughts and promote a good night's sleep. These oils contain antidepressant, sedative, and irritability-reducing properties.

Yield: ¼ cup

RECIPE
9 drops vetiver oil
3 drops lavender oil
3 drops geranium oil
¼ cup cornstarch

Place the ingredients into a mason jar, stirring well with a whisk. Carefully poke holes into the lid, use this as a shaker, and shake the ingredients into pillowcases or under sheet areas as needed. You can get a piece of plastic wrap and place it over the jar and under the lid to keep powder from spilling out when not in use. Store in a glass jar or container with a tight-fitting lid in a cool, dark, and dry area for up to 3 months.

Relaxing Flowers Bath Salts

This essential oil recipe is great to help a person unwind after a stressful day with its analgesic, anti-inflammatory, sedative, and antidepressant properties. Relax and get rid of those troubling thoughts.

Yield: 3 cups

RECIPE
7 drops patchouli oil
7 drops cypress oil
7 drops geranium oil
3 drops vitamin E oil
2 tablespoons carrier oil
3 cups salts
1 tablespoon milk (optional for adults, recommended for children)

Use any type of salt you prefer: pink Himalayan salt, sea salt, Epsom salts, etc. In a small container, add the essential oils to the desired type of salt. Stir until well blended. Screw lid onto container tightly. Leave mixture in a dark area for 24 hours and then stir mixture again. Run the bathwater. Once the tub is full of water, you can add the milk, and then add ½ cup of the bath salt mixture to bathwater as you get into the tub. You may stay in the tub as long as the temperature is comfortable. Dry your feet well when you get out of the bath, as the oils are slippery and can cause you to fall. Store remainder in a glass jar or container with a tight-fitting lid in a cool, dark area for up to 3 months. These jars make attractive, inexpensive, and healing gifts!

One Foot at a Time Rub

This recipe contains a powerful blend of oils to help you to remain calm and reestablish your focus where it needs to be, rather than obsessively mull over the thoughts that trouble you. The therapeutic properties at work in this recipe include tonic, antidepressant, and sedative components.

Yield: 1–2 applications

RECIPE
1 drop lavender oil
1 drop vetiver oil
1 drop frankincense oil
2 drops vitamin E oil
1 tablespoon carrier oil

Pour the essential oils, carrier oil, and any remaining ingredients into a small glass container, bowl, or jar. Swirl or whisk to mix the ingredients and apply lightly to the area desired, such as pressure points, neck, soles of feet, temples, or chest. Keep essential oil mixture away from open wounds, mucus membranes, genitals, eyes, and sensitive areas. Repeat application as needed, usually 2–3 times daily. You may cover area with linen or cloth to protect clothing and furniture. Store unused portion in a glass jar or container with a tight-fitting lid in a cool, dark area for up to 3 months.

Pain

Sensory neurons in our brain receive messages from all parts of our body that relay comfort or discomfort. Pain can range from mild and annoying to pure agony. Ridding the body of pain is a priority among most people. Numerous methods have been used for centuries to rid one of pain, but plants, trees, and herbs were always thought to be among the best options for people. Essential oils are the essences of those plants. Many essential oils contain therapeutic properties that combat pain and bring peace to the body. The following essential oils all contain analgesic and anti-inflammatory agents along with properties that will reduce pain significantly.

Essential Oils

Chamomile, clary sage, clove, eucalyptus, fennel, fir, frankincense, ginger, helichrysum, lavender, marjoram, peppermint, Roman chamomile, rosemary, sandalwood, spruce, thyme, vetiver, wintergreen, and yarrow

Murmuring Muscle Rub

Pain from arthritis, bones, muscles, and deep aches can be relieved with this blend of essential oils. Rub this mixture in deep over the site of pain and within minutes your pain may decrease and you can carry on with your day.

Yield: 1 fluid ounce

RECIPE

9 drops helichrysum oil

5 drops juniper oil

5 drops marjoram oil

4 drops chamomile oil

4 drops vitamin E oil

1 fluid ounce carrier oil

Pour the essential oils, carrier oil, and any remaining ingredients into a small glass container, bowl, or jar. Swirl or whisk to mix the ingredients, apply lightly, and rub in to the area desired, such joints, bones and muscles. Keep essential oil mixture away from open wounds, mucus membranes, genitals, eyes, and sensitive areas. Repeat application as needed, usually 2–3 times daily. You may cover area with linen or cloth to protect clothing and furniture. Store unused portion in a glass jar or container with a tight-fitting lid in a cool, dark area for up to 3 months.

Soothing Balm

This balm is great for foot pain, lower back pain, and most localized pains. The essential oils in this recipe have analgesic and anti-inflammatory properties to help with quieting that pain so you can relax and enjoy yourself.

Yield: 2 tablespoons

RECIPE
3 drops peppermint oil
3 drops vetiver oil
3 drops frankincense oil
3 drops thyme oil
1 tablespoon carrier oil
½ teaspoon beeswax pellets
4 drops vitamin E oil

Heat the beeswax and the carrier oil in a glass bowl in the microwave for 1½–2 minutes, until just melted, or on low on the stovetop. If you open the door every 15 seconds, you can avoid the popping of the wax and oil and overheating. Carefully remove the container from the microwave and stir. Drip a drop of the melted oil and wax onto the counter, after 1 minute check for consistency. If it is too thin, add more beeswax to the container; if it is too thick, add more carrier oil. Add the vitamin E oil and the essential oil to the heated mixture in the container. Whisk lightly, and it will begin hardening immediately. Pour into containers. Ensure your containers are glass or tin to prevent leeching of chemicals. Once cool, apply a thin coating to the painful areas on your body. Do not apply to mucus membranes, eyes, genitals, or open wounds. Label containers and store in a dark, dry area for up to 1 year.

San-Zen Wrap

This wrap is great for healing elbows, knees, ankles, and any area you can wrap with a piece of linen, gauze, or bandage and leave it in place for a while. These essential oils not only have pain-relieving therapeutic properties, but they smell great too! I love to use this wrap on my achy bones and muscles when I am just going to be sitting still for a period of time.

Yield: 1 application

RECIPE
3 drops lavender oil
3 drops ginger oil
2 drops chamomile oil
2 drops juniper oil
2 drops spruce oil
1 tablespoon carrier oil
1 piece muslin or linen

Mix ingredients together into a small bowl or container. Apply the mixture onto a long, rectangle piece of muslin, linen, gauze, or cotton. Wrap the treated material around the wrist, knee, ankle, etc. Leave for at least 15 minutes. Store remainder of ingredients in a container with a tight-fitting lid for up to 30 days.

Panic Attacks

A person suffering panic attacks often feels as if they are dying. The attack can manifest itself in many different ways, for many different reasons. Getting the person calm is the number one goal during the attack. If you or someone you know feels that they are about to have a panic attack, using one of these oils can help to lessen the anxious and fearful feelings associated with panic attacks. Essential oils can help with calming a person down, and for preventing further attacks.

Essential Oils

Frankincense, lavender, lemon, linden blossom, rosemary, and ylang-ylang

Panic Reducing Hand Rub

The essential oils in this blend work wonderfully together to bring a sense of calm and confidence to the wearer. Not only does it relax you, but the aromas linger and envelop you with a sense of comfort.

Yield: 1–2 applications

RECIPE

3 drops lavender oil

3 drops frankincense oil

2 drops linden blossom oil

2 drops vitamin E oil (optional)

Enough warm water to fill bowl halfway

Combine the ingredients together into a small bowl. Dip one hand into the bowl until fingers are covered in the oils. Rub hands together for 5–15 minutes, rinse if desired, and repeat as often as needed. Ensure that the oils have been completely absorbed into your skin before touching furniture, clothing, etc., or oils may stain. I sometimes wear gloves throughout the night over the oils to ensure that the therapeutic properties are absorbed to their fullest all night long. Pour remainder into a jar with a tight-fitting lid, and store in a cool, dark area for up to 1 month.

Beautiful Breath Powder

If suffering from panic attacks, anxiety, or night terrors, this powder, when placed inside the pillowcases and under the sheets, can bring a night full of peace and deep sleep. The slumber and peace-inducing essential oils contain analgesic, sedative, hypotensive, and nervine properties.

Yield: ¼ cup

RECIPE

3 drops lavender oil

3 drops frankincense oil

3 drops linden blossom oil

4 drops vitamin E oil

¼ cup cornstarch

Place the ingredients into a mason jar, stirring well with a whisk. Carefully poke holes into the lid, use this as a shaker, and shake the ingredients into pillowcases or under sheet areas as needed. You can get a piece of plastic wrap and place it over the jar and under the lid to keep powder from spilling out when not in use. Store in a glass jar or container with a tight-fitting lid in a cool, dark, and dry area for up to 3 months.

Calming Aromas Bath Salts

These bath salts contain essential oils that are calming and soothing and will help a person gain strength from their inner selves to help control chaotic thoughts. This positivity-inducing and calming bath is perfect for someone prone to panic attacks. The essential oils in this recipe include hypotensive, antidepressant, and nervine properties.

Yield: 3 cups

RECIPE

7 drops rosemary oil

7 drops linden blossom oil

7 drops ylang-ylang oil

2 tablespoons carrier oil

4 drops vitamin E oil

3 cups salts

1 tablespoon milk (optional for adults, recommended for children)

Use any type of salt you prefer: pink Himalayan salt, sea salt, Epsom salts, etc. In a small container, add the essential oils to the desired type of salt. Stir until well blended. Screw lid onto container tightly. Leave mixture in a dark area for 24 hours and then stir mixture again. Run the bathwater. Once the tub is full of water, you can add the milk, and then add ½ cup of the bath salt mixture to bathwater as you get into the tub. You may stay in the tub as long as the temperature is comfortable. Dry your feet well when you get out of the bath, as the oils are slippery and can cause you to fall. Store remainder in a glass jar or container with a tight-fitting lid in a cool, dark area for up to 3 months. These jars make attractive, inexpensive, and healing gifts!

End the Hell Inhale

Persons suffering from panic attacks feel that they are not able to go into public for fear of having an attack. Carry these essential oils in your purse or car, and you will be able to ward off an attack by inhaling the smell of these oils at the first sign of stress. Each of these oils contains detoxifying and analgesic properties.

Yield: 1 application

RECIPE
1 drop lemon oil

or

1 drop frankincense oil

Choose your essential oil and apply to the palm of your hand, an oil inhaler, or a tissue. Bring the essential oils close to your nostrils and inhale the aroma deeply. You can cover one nostril at a time with your thumb and, if you prefer, alternate nostrils. This process sends the properties straight to your brain and the effects are immediate. You can complete this procedure 3–4 times daily.

Paranoia

The thought processes that wrongly lead a person to believe that others are out to get him or her is often diagnosed as paranoia. Irrational fear and a feeling of conspiracy against them is a common theme in someone suffering from paranoia. There are many illnesses and diseases that can cause a person to have these feelings and delusions. Mental health professionals should be enlisted in the event of chronic paranoia. Many medications are on the market today that can curb these feelings of unease, danger, and threat. Essential oils have been known to calm a person and assist them in having more rational thought processes and have been used for this purpose for hundreds of years.

Essential Oils

Basil, bergamot, cassia, citrus, cypress, frankincense, geranium, lavender, lemon, lime, melissa, rosewood, sandalwood, vetiver, and ylang-ylang

Paranoia Linen Powder

This recipe has powerful, calming essential oils to bring one's mind back to focus. Putting a little of this under the sheets can have a person calmly falling into a deep slumber, instead of spending the night in a constant state of hyperawareness. The calming ingredients in this recipe contain antidepressant, aphrodisiac, nervine, and sedative properties, among others.

Yield: ¼ cup

RECIPE

3 drops lavender oil

3 drops ylang-ylang oil

3 drops orange oil

4 drops vitamin E oil

¼ cup cornstarch

Place the ingredients into a mason jar, stirring well with a whisk. Carefully poke holes into the lid, use this as a shaker, and shake the ingredients into pillowcases or under sheet areas as needed. You can get a piece of plastic wrap and place it over the jar and under the lid to keep powder from spilling out when not in use. Store in a glass jar or container with a tight-fitting lid in a cool, dark, and dry area for up to 3 months.

Beautiful World Bath Salts

These bath salts won't allow fear to overtake you, but a peaceful bliss with delightful aromas will invade your senses. So relax into this bath and concentrate on how lucky you are to live in this beautiful world. The therapeutic properties in this blend include antidepressant, sedative, and tranquilizing agents.

Yield: 3 cups

RECIPE

5 drops vetiver oil

5 drops bergamot oil

5 drops rosewood oil

5 drops orange oil

5 drops vitamin E oil

2 tablespoons carrier oil

3 cups salts

Use any type of salt you prefer: pink Himalayan salt, sea salt, Epsom salts, etc. In a small container, add the essential oils to the desired type of salt. Stir until well blended. Screw lid onto container tightly. Leave mixture in a dark area for 24 hours and then stir mixture again. Run the bathwater. Once the tub is full of water, you can add the milk, and then add ½ cup of the bath salt mixture to bathwater as you get into the tub. You may stay in the tub as long as the temperature is comfortable. Dry your feet well when you get out of the bath, as the oils are slippery and can cause you to fall. Store remainder in a glass jar or container with a tight-fitting lid in a cool, dark area for up to 3 months. These jars make attractive, inexpensive, and healing gifts!

No Fear Rub

This blend of essential oils rubbed on the temples, neck, and chest can calm even the most agitated and paranoid of people! So, if your loved one is having negative thoughts about others turning against them, then getting a little massage with this blend will be just what they need to bring their thoughts back down to earth. The calming properties are antidepressant, restorative, nerve-relieving, and sedative.

Yield: 1 tablespoon

RECIPE

2 drops cypress oil

2 drops basil oil

2 drops lavender oil

2 drops vitamin E oil

1 tablespoon carrier oil

Pour the essential oils, carrier oil, and any remaining ingredients into a small glass container, bowl, or jar. Swirl or whisk to mix the ingredients and apply lightly to the area desired, such as pressure points, neck, soles of feet, temples, or chest. Keep essential oil mixture away from open wounds, mucus membranes, genitals, eyes, and sensitive areas. Repeat application as needed, usually 2–3 times daily. You may cover area with linen or cloth to protect clothing and furniture. Store unused portion in a glass jar or container with a tight-fitting lid in a cool, dark area for up to 3 months.

Enchanting Thoughts Air

This diffuser blend is a relaxing, peaceful way to curb those negative thought processes. Let the peace and gratitude take over your home, as well as the delightful aromas imparted by this recipe. This aromatic blend contains antidepressant, aphrodisiac, calming, sedative, and tonic properties.

Yield: 1 application

RECIPE
4 drops rosewood oil
1 drop cassia oil
2 drops sandalwood oil
Water

Follow your directions for using essential oils in your particular brand of diffuser. Ensure that your diffuser does not use heat but runs by vibration, sound waves, or another cold-steam type of process. Choose the essential oils needed for your condition, then add water and oils to the diffuser. Run your diffuser as needed to permeate the air with therapeutic properties and achieve the results you desire.

Just Chillin' Compress

This compress will have you just chillin' and relaxin' in no time. If you have a family member who is constantly agitated and in a place of fear, this compress will relax them and let peaceful thoughts saturate their brain instead of worries and stress. This blend contains antidepressant, aphrodisiac, sedative, and tranquilizing properties.

Yield: 1 application

RECIPE
2 drops frankincense oil

2 drops vetiver oil

4 drops vitamin E oil

1 wet cloth

Fold a long piece of cloth (muslin, linen, or gauze) into a rectangle. Wet the cloth and wring out very well. In the center of the cloth, apply a mixture of the blended oils. Wrap the cloth around the area desired and leave on for approximately 15 minutes, or as long as comfortable. When done, wash cloth for re-use. Apply 3–4 times daily until desired effects are achieved.

Deep Thoughts Massage

Relaxing and calming the thought process can take a person from paranoia to peacefulness. These essential oils will go deep into the cells and help bring comfort. It is such a calming and aromatic massage that the person giving the massage will feel relaxed as well! The essential oils in this recipe contain tranquilizing, sedative, antidepressant and aphrodisiac properties.

Yield: 1 fluid ounce

RECIPE

10 drops vetiver oil

4 drops geranium oil

4 drops ylang-ylang oil

3 drops vitamin E oil

1 fluid ounce carrier oil

Pour the essential oils and the carrier oil into a small glass container, bowl, or jar. Swirl to mix the ingredients and use to massage lightly the area desired, such as temples, neck, chest, back, or soles of feet. Keep essential oil mixture away from open wounds, mucus membranes, genitals, eyes, and sensitive areas. Repeat application as needed. Store unused portion in a glass jar or container with a tight-fitting lid in a cool, dark area for up to 3 months.

Heavenly Inhale

Carry a vial of one of these oils with you at all times so that you can feel calm at a moment's notice. Help to rid yourself of all anxiety and enjoy your surroundings. These essential oils contain calming, sedative, and nervine properties.

Yield: 1 application

RECIPE
1 drop lavender oil

or

1 drop vetiver oil

or

1 drop basil oil

Choose your essential oil and apply to the palm of your hand, an oil inhaler, or a tissue. Bring the essential oils close to your nostrils and inhale the aroma deeply. You can cover one nostril at a time with your thumb and, if you prefer, alternate nostrils. This process sends the properties straight to your brain and the effects are immediate. You can complete this procedure 3–4 times daily.

Be Calm Bath

A great morning bath that uses the essential oils to energize you but keeps you focused and peaceful at the same time. This balancing blend contains antidepressant, aphrodisiac, tonic, and sedative properties.

Yield: 1 application

RECIPE
5 drops orange oil
5 drops melissa oil
5 drops cypress oil
1 tablespoon carrier oil
1 tablespoon milk (optional for adults, recommended for children)

As you begin to fill the tub with water, pour the chosen essential oils and carrier oil into the running water. Run a warm, not hot, bath. Water that is too hot will cause the essential oils to dissipate. You may add 1 tablespoon of milk to the water; this ensures that the essential oils will not stick to your skin, but will mix with the water. You may soak in the water as long as you are comfortable. Dry your feet well once you get out of the water, as the oils will cause them to be slippery, increasing your chances of falling. Rinse the tub of any remaining oils.

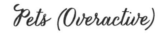

Pets (Overactive)

Sometimes a pet can become stressed, overactive, and unruly due to external factors. Making a spray with essential oils and lightly spraying onto your pet's fur can help them to calm down, de-stress, and relax for a time. Some essential oils are extremely dangerous for pets, so ensure that you read all warnings on your essential oil labels regarding pets.

Essential Oils

Chamomile, lavender, mandarin, marjoram, and orange

Pet Calming Spray

This pet spray works so well for my Silkie when she is overly agitated and unable to sleep due to changes in the home, such as company staying the night or a trip to the vet. She will just lie down and have the best night's sleep after a quick spray of this on her back. This blend contains antidepressant, sedative, and tranquilizing properties.

Yield: 2 fluid ounces

RECIPE
4 drops lavender oil
4 drops chamomile oil
4 drops mandarin oil
1 tablespoon apple cider vinegar
2 fluid ounces water

Add all ingredients to a dark-colored spray bottle. Check for material steadfastness before spraying on fabric. Shake bottle and spray onto back, lightly. Do not spray into or on open wounds, genitals, eyes, or mucus membranes. Store in a cool, dark area for up to 3 months. Shake well before each use to combine the ingredients.

Good Smell Spray

When your dog rolls around in poop, dead frogs, or other stinky messes, this is the spray I use if I don't have time to give mine a bath. This blend smells so good, yet also has calming, sedative, and tranquilizing properties to help pets calm down and go with the flow.

Yield: 2 fluid ounces

RECIPE

5 drops lavender oil

5 drops orange oil

10 drops mandarin oil

1 tablespoon apple cider vinegar

2 fluid ounces water

Add all ingredients to a dark-colored spray bottle. Check for material steadfastness before spraying on fabric. Shake bottle and spray lightly onto back. Do not spray into or on open wounds, genitals, eyes, or mucus membranes. Store in a cool, dark area for up to 3 months. Shake well before each use to combine the ingredients.

Doggie's Room Spray

This spray works beautifully for ridding the home of a dog's odors. The house always smells wonderful due to the antiseptic properties in this blend.

Yield: 2 fluid ounces

RECIPE

5 drops mandarin oil

5 drops orange oil

5 drops lavender oil

1 tablespoon apple cider vinegar

2 fluid ounces water

Add all ingredients to a dark-colored spray bottle. Check for material steadfastness before spraying on fabric. Shake bottle and spray lightly onto back. Do not spray into or on open wounds, genitals, eyes, or mucus membranes. Store in a cool, dark area for up to 3 months. Shake well before each use to combine the ingredients.

Rejection

Healing from rejection can be achieved over a period of time. Essential oils can help with that healing by bringing calming, uplifting, forgiving, and self-loving properties that we can use daily to end those feelings of rejection. These oils have been used for many centuries to heal broken hearts or broken trust and replace those feelings with empowerment.

Essential Oils

Bay laurel, bergamot, cedarwood, eucalyptus, frankincense, helichrysum, jasmine, lemon, marjoram, myrrh, pine, Roman chamomile, and rose

Reject that Rejection Hand Rub

Not only do the therapeutic properties in this recipe bring comfort to your soul, but the rubbing motion on your hands helps to calm and soothe you.

Yield: 1–2 applications

RECIPE
3 drops Roman chamomile oil
3 drops rose oil
2 drops jasmine oil
2 drops vitamin E oil (optional)
Enough warm water to fill bowl halfway

Combine the ingredients together into a small bowl. Dip one hand into the bowl until fingers are covered in the oils. Rub hands together for 5–15 minutes, rinse if desired, and repeat as often as needed. Ensure that the oils have been completely absorbed into your skin before touching furniture, clothing, etc., or oils may stain. I sometimes wear gloves throughout the night over the oils to ensure that the therapeutic properties are absorbed to their fullest all night long. Pour remainder into a jar with a tight-fitting lid, and store in a cool, dark area for up to 1 month.

Inward Reflection Spray

This spray has uplifting essential oils in it that will help you to focus on the positive and stay away from the negative. Our inner thoughts can drive us to insanity and make us take certain actions that we will regret. When your feelings are hurt by rejection and betrayal, it takes effort to repair yourself. These essential oils can help to show you the bright side of life and leave the sadness behind.

Yield: 2 fluid ounces

RECIPE
10 drops lemon oil
5 drops helichrysum oil
5 drops frankincense oil
1 tablespoon witch hazel
2 fluid ounces water

Add all ingredients to a dark-colored spray bottle. Check for material steadfastness before spraying on fabric. Shake the bottle and spray onto area desired, such as body, hair, home, car, or office. Do not spray into or on open wounds, genitals, eyes, or mucus membranes. Store in a cool, dark area for up to 3 months. Shake well before each use to combine the ingredients.

Soul Balm

This salve has essential oils that provide healing for a broken spirit due to rejection or betrayal. A balm for the soul is necessary to get through the grieving process and begin to have faith in humanity again. These oils are derived from plants that were used as far back as medieval times to heal people who had been betrayed and rejected by friends, loved ones, and lovers.

Yield: 1 tablespoon

RECIPE

7 drops rose oil

5 drops jasmine oil

3 drops bay laurel oil

1 teaspoon beeswax pellets

4 drops vitamin E oil

3 teaspoons carrier oil

Heat the beeswax and the carrier oil in a glass bowl in the microwave for 1½–2 minutes, until just melted, or on low on the stovetop. If you open the door every 15 seconds, you can avoid the popping of the wax and oil and overheating. Carefully remove the container from the microwave and stir. Drip a drop of the melted oil and wax onto the counter, after 1 minute check for consistency. If it is too thin, add more beeswax to the container; if it is too thick, add more carrier oil. Add the vitamin E oil and the essential oil to the heated mixture in the container. Whisk lightly, and it will begin hardening immediately. Pour into containers. Ensure your containers are glass or tin to prevent leeching of chemicals. Once cool, apply to wrists, temples, neck, or soles of feet. Do not apply to mucus membranes, eyes, genitals, or open wounds. Label containers and store in a dark, dry area for up to 1 year.

Blow 'Em Away Bombs

Your mood can't help but to be lifted by using one of these bath and shower bombs in your tub. Not only do the fizzing and the aromas of the bombs help to relax and comfort you, but the essential oils are full of properties to help you to start the forgiving process that is needed for true healing and to open your heart, loving the person that you are again.

Yield: 8–12 bombs

RECIPE

1 cup baking soda

½ cup citric acid

½ cup cornstarch

½ cup Epsom salts, fine grained

15 drops chamomile oil

15 drops bergamot oil

10 drops myrrh oil

½ teaspoon carrier oil

¾ teaspoon water

spray bottle (water)

In a large bowl, mix your dry ingredients together until fine with a whisk. In a tiny jar with a lid, add your wet ingredients and shake to mix. You may add a couple drops of food coloring to the wet jar. Extremely slowly, add the wet ingredients to the dry ingredients while whisking rapidly. If fizzing takes place, whisk until it is mixed. Once the ingredients are well mixed, it should be the texture of slightly damp sand. Add a spray or two of water if needed. Once the mixture is the consistency you like, form into balls; I just smash mine down into ice cube trays or muffin tins. You can use cute molds, but you must work rapidly as mixture will dry out quickly. Leave in open air, uncovered, in a room where they will not be disturbed for 12–24 hours. Once they are dry, you can place 1–2 bombs into your bath or directly into the spray of the shower and they will fizz and release their aromatic and healing properties. Store unused portion in an airtight container for up to 6 months.

Low Self-Esteem

Low self-esteem can be summed up as not believing in yourself. We often, through childhood, nurture, or nature, do not develop the self-love that we need to enjoy our successes in life or to even think that we deserve the successes that we have achieved. We do not have confidence in ourselves or our abilities to complete a project, speak out loud, look people in the eyes, or any number of things that a lot of people do instinctually. These essential oils will help a person with their self-assurance, self-impressions, and self-regard.

Essential Oils

Basil, bergamot, chamomile, elemi, fennel, frankincense, geranium, jasmine, melissa, myrrh, neroli, rose, rosemary, rosewood, sandalwood, spruce, vetiver, and ylang-ylang

Wear It like a Boss

This laundry detergent has essential oils in it that contain agents known to help a person to boost their confidence, and it smells great, too. It has properties that work to lessen anxiety and calm a person, while at the same time instilling a sense of confidence and joy. I have listed men's and women's fragrances separately, but anyone can wear either one!

Yield: ¼ cup

RECIPE

(Men)
3 drops spruce oil
3 drops frankincense oil
¼ cup unscented liquid laundry detergent

Mix the ingredients together in a small bowl or container. Stir well. Add the manufacturer's recommended amount of oil-infused laundry detergent to each load in the washer. Store remainder in a glass jar with a tight-fitting lid in a cool, dark area for up to 1 year.

(Women)
2 drops rosewood oil
2 drops melissa oil
1 drop neroli oil
¼ cup unscented liquid laundry detergent

Mix the ingredients together in a small bowl or container. Stir well. Add the manufacturer's recommended amount of detergent to each load in the washer. Store remainder in a glass jar with a tight-fitting lid in a cool, dark area for up to 1 year.

Bomb Splash

This recipe has essential oils that can permeate your brain with self-love and bolster your confidence enough that you can get through anything. Luxuriate in this bath and inhale the aromas that waft through your self-made, spa-like retreat. When you climb out of the tub, not only will you feel like you may be able to speak before a crowd of thousands, but you will have the oils clinging to every pore in your body and exuding their properties into your system the entire day and night.

Yield: 8–12 bombs

RECIPE

1 cup baking soda

½ cup citric acid

½ cup cornstarch

½ cup Epsom salts, fine grained

15 drops vetiver oil

15 drops sandalwood oil

5 drops jasmine oil

½ teaspoon carrier oil

¾ teaspoon water

spray bottle (water)

In a large bowl, mix your dry ingredients together until fine with a whisk. In a tiny jar with a lid, add your wet ingredients and shake to mix. You may add a couple drops of food coloring to the wet jar. Extremely slowly, add the wet ingredients to the dry ingredients while whisking rapidly. If fizzing takes place, whisk until it is mixed. Once the ingredients are well mixed, it should be the texture of slightly damp sand. Add a spray or two of water if needed. Once the mixture is the consistency you like, form into balls; I just smash mine down into ice cube trays or muffin tins. You can use cute molds, but you must work rapidly as mixture will dry out quickly. Leave in open air, uncovered, in a room where they will not be disturbed for 12–24 hours. Once they are dry, you can place 1–2 bombs into your bath or directly into the spray of the shower and they will fizz and release their aromatic and healing properties. Store unused portion in an airtight container for up to 6 months.

Self-Esteem Lip Balm

Use this wonderfully hydrating lip balm the next time you want to give yourself that added little boost of self-esteem. Moisturizing and full of healing oils, this balm not only makes you feel better, but its healing properties will help your lips look their best.

Yield: 1 tablespoon

RECIPE

3 teaspoons grape seed oil

½ teaspoon beeswax pellets

4 drops vitamin E oil

3 drops rose oil

3 drops pink melissa oil

Melt the beeswax and the carrier oil in a glass bowl in the microwave until most of the beeswax is melted. You can also use a pan on the stovetop on low. Cool slightly. Add the vitamin E and the essential oils and stir or whisk quickly. With a spoon, drip a drop of the mixture onto the counter and Let set for 1 minute. Pull your finger through the drop and check for consistency. If mixture is too thin, add more beeswax; if it is too thick, add more oil. Once desired consistency is acquired, immediately pour into small balm container (glass or metal) with a lid. After mixture cools, cover and store in a cool, dark area for up to 6 months.

Worry

Worry is the constant repetition of thoughts about an anticipated event or potential problem. Many people suffer from constant worry; it interrupts their sleeping process, causes mood changes, and adds stress to their body, causing illness. My mantra when I start worrying is to say to myself, "What's the worst that can happen?" I envision the worst, then envision the best possible outcome. I try to focus on the best outcome and try to keep my thoughts pointed in that direction. The following blends use essential oils reputed to calm the mind and help turn negative thoughts to positive thoughts.

Essential Oils

Basil, bay laurel, bergamot, chamomile, clary sage, coriander, eucalyptus, frankincense, jasmine, lemon, lime, magnolia, marjoram, melissa, neroli, patchouli, pine, sandalwood, spikenard, spruce, tangerine, valerian, vanilla, vetiver, wild orange, and ylang-ylang

What's the Worst That Can Happen Temple Rub

I like to use this rub to help ease my tormenting of myself with overthinking and to bring calm to my overactive thoughts. Not only do the calming therapeutic properties in this blend help to dispel worry, but the circular motion on my temples eases my mind and spirit.

Yield: 1 tablespoon

RECIPE

3 drops bay laurel oil

3 drops tangerine oil

1 drop vanilla oil

1 tablespoon carrier oil

Pour the essential oils, carrier oil, and any remaining ingredients into a small glass container, bowl, or jar. Swirl or whisk to mix the ingredients and apply lightly to the area desired, such as temples or neck. Keep essential oil mixture away from open wounds, mucus membranes, genitals, eyes, and sensitive areas. Repeat application as needed, usually 2–3 times daily. You may cover area with linen or cloth to protect clothing and furniture. Store unused portion in a glass jar or container with a tight-fitting lid in a cool, dark area for up to 3 months.

Thoughtless Sleep Linen Spray

I keep a little bottle of this linen spray by my bed to use on those nights of mental distress and it will bring me peace, relief, and sometimes smiles. The weeks of the full moon are the worst for worriers. Plan ahead and spray the bed! Calming and sedative properties work in this blend to reduce anxiety and promote a good night's sleep.

Yield: 2 fluid ounces

RECIPE

5 drops vetiver oil

5 drops spikenard oil

5 drops valerian oil

1 fluid ounce distilled water

1 fluid ounce vodka

Add all ingredients to a dark-colored spray bottle. Check for material steadfastness before spraying on fabric. Shake the bottle and spray onto area desired, such as body, hair, home, car, or office. Do not spray into or on open wounds, genitals, eyes, or mucus membranes. Store in a cool, dark area for up to 3 months. Shake well before each use to combine the ingredients.

It's a Good Day

When you find yourself worrying about an upcoming meeting and getting yourself worked up with apprehension about potential problems that could happen, just inhale a little of one of these aromas to bring your thoughts back down to earth, reduce anxiety, and impart a sense of peace and calm to any situation.

Yield: 1 application

RECIPE

1 drop melissa oil

or

1 drop wild orange oil

or

1 drop magnolia oil

Choose your essential oil and apply to the palm of your hand, an oil inhaler, or a tissue. Bring the essential oils close to your nostrils and inhale the aroma deeply. You can cover one nostril at a time with your thumb and, if you prefer, alternate nostrils. This process sends the properties straight to your brain and the effects are immediate. You can complete this procedure 3–4 times daily.

CHAPTER 4
Recipes for Emotions

There are more emotions in you than can even be named. You can feel complete bliss and joy at the simple smile of an infant, or utter devastation by the expression on a friend's face. Some emotions are sought after for a lifetime; some are unwanted and seem to always be lurking in the shadows. Essential oils have been proven time and again to help you to achieve the emotions you desire and curb the emotions that plague you. For thousands of years cultures all over the earth have used essential oils to help control emotional needs.

The skin is a very good conductor of essential oils. Science has shown that within seconds of applying essential oils to the soles of the feet or to other areas of the body, every cell within you has evidence of that oil being present. These cells transport the therapeutic properties of these oils to the areas of the brain responsible for emotions, giving us peace, calm, relaxation, energy, and a myriad of other boosts to portions of our emotional selves.

Always heed the warnings listed in the back of this book and follow the tips at the beginning. You will find that using essential oils is fun, beneficial, and can bring harmony and happiness at a moment's notice.

Agitation

You know that feeling when you're not quite angry, but you're extremely annoyed, and the feeling persists throughout the day with everything you do and everyone you meet? That's being agitated and the causes of agitation are numerous. Calming and relaxing essential oils can have you feeling peaceful and grounded again in no time at all.

Essential Oils

Bergamot, dill, cedarwood, chamomile, eucalyptus, frankincense, jasmine, lavender, lemon, neroli, orange, Palo Santo, patchouli, peppermint, petitgrain, Roman chamomile, rose, sandalwood, tea tree, and vetiver

Balm Bomb

Apply these essential oils and blast that agitated feeling to smithereens. When every little sentence out of my husband's mouth makes me roll my eyes in agitation, I bring out the balm bomb to soothe my spirit and soul and make me smile instead of get all tight-lipped toward him. These calming and healing therapeutic properties will ground you and have you smiling in no time.

Yield: 1 fluid ounce

RECIPE
1 fluid ounce carrier oil
1–s beeswax pellets
4 drops vitamin E oil
6 drops lavender oil
6 drops bergamot oil
6 drops sandalwood oil

Heat the beeswax and the carrier oil in a glass bowl in the microwave for 1½–2 minutes, until just melted, or on low on the stovetop. If you open the door every 15 seconds, you can avoid the popping of the wax and oil and overheating. Carefully remove the container from the microwave and stir. Drip a drop of the melted oil and wax onto the counter, and after 1 minute check for consistency. If it is too thin, add more beeswax to the container; if it is too thick, add more carrier oil. Add the vitamin E oil and the essential oil to the heated mixture in the container. Whisk lightly, and it will begin hardening immediately. Pour into containers. Ensure your containers are glass or tin to prevent leeching of chemicals. Once cool, apply to wrists, temples, neck, or soles of feet. Do not apply to mucus membranes, eyes, genitals, or open wounds. Label containers and store in a dark, dry area for up to 1 year.

Fingers of Calm

This little hand rub recipe has the power to banish negative energy and replace it with positive energy. Let your hands absorb these oils and every time you get them near your face, the calming and happy feelings from inhaling the properties will flood you and you won't feel agitated anymore. The hands are great conductors of essential oils into the body and straight to the brain, which fills you with the positive healing benefits of this blend.

Yield: ½ ounce

RECIPE
3 drops Palo Santo oil
3 drops rose oil
3 drops petitgrain oil
½ ounce carrier oil
4 drops vitamin E oil

Combine the ingredients together into a small bowl. Dip one hand into the bowl until fingers are covered in the oils. Rub hands together for 5–15 minutes, rinse if desired, and repeat as often as needed. Ensure that the oils have been completely absorbed into your skin before touching furniture, clothing, etc., or oils may stain. I sometimes wear gloves throughout the night over the oils to ensure that the therapeutic properties are absorbed to their fullest all night long. Pour remainder into a jar with a tight-fitting lid, and store in a cool, dark area for up to 1 month.

Relax That Jaw

When stress, tension, and agitation are present, we tend to clench our jaws and teeth. This diffuser will help you to relax your muscles, thereby reducing your agitation and stress. I love the effects and aromas of these oils in a diffuser and run them often.

Yield: 1 application

RECIPE
5 drops frankincense oil
5 drops neroli oil
5 drops cedarwood oil
Water

Follow your directions for using essential oils in your particular brand of diffuser. Ensure that your diffuser does not use heat but runs by vibration, sound waves, or another cold-steam type of process. Choose the essential oils needed for your condition, then add water and oils to the diffuser. Run your diffuser as needed to permeate the air with therapeutic properties and achieve the results you desire. This blend will allow you to receive the desired effect, reduce agitation, and relax that jaw.

Agitation Salve

This blend will soothe even the most agitated spirit. The therapeutic properties in this salve work together to provide the wearer with calm and tranquil thoughts.

Yield: 1 tablespoon

RECIPE
7 drops rose oil
5 drops vetiver oil
3 drops tea tree (melaleuca) oil
1 teaspoon beeswax pellets
4 drops vitamin E oil
3 teaspoons carrier oil

Heat the beeswax and the carrier oil in a glass bowl in the microwave for 1 ½–2 minutes, until just melted, or on low on the stovetop. If you open the door every 15 seconds, you can avoid the popping of the wax and oil and overheating. Carefully remove the container from the microwave and stir. Drip a drop of the melted oil and wax onto the counter, after 1 minute check for consistency. If it is too thin, add more beeswax to the container; if it is too thick, add more carrier oil. Add the vitamin E oil and the essential oil to the heated mixture in the container. Whisk lightly, and it will begin hardening immediately. Pour into containers. Ensure your containers are glass or tin to prevent leeching of chemicals. Once cool, apply to wrists, temples, neck, or soles of feet. Do not apply to mucus membranes, eyes, genitals, or open wounds. Label containers and store in a dark, dry area for up to 1 year.

Anger

Anger is a reaction to a perceived threat. The blood pressure rises and adrenaline courses through the body. When one has anger responses to too many situations, then stress, strife, and illness soon follow. Essential oils are well known to assuage a person's anger and bring calmness. Diet, exercise, and meditation are also inexpensive or free and great for helping a person to learn to control their attitudes and responses toward others.

Essential Oils

Benzoin, bergamot, chamomile, clary sage, geranium, grapefruit, lavender, myrrh, patchouli, peppermint, sandalwood, spearmint, vetiver, and ylang-ylang

Calming Powder

This powder, sprinkled under the sheets, will help you keep true to that old adage we try to follow of "never going to bed angry." Some of the calming and peaceful properties of these essential oils are harmonizing, sedative, nervine, antidepressant, detoxifying, restorative, and tonic.

Yield: ¼ cup

Recipe

3 drops lavender oil

3 drops clary sage oil

3 drops sandalwood oil

¼ cup cornstarch

4 drops vitamin E oil

Place the ingredients into a mason jar, stirring well with a whisk. Carefully poke holes into the lid, use this as a shaker, and shake the ingredients into pillowcases or under sheet areas as needed. You can get a piece of plastic wrap and place it over the jar and under the lid to keep powder from spilling out when not in use. Store in a glass jar or container with a tight-fitting lid in a cool, dark, and dry area for up to 3 months.

Mellow Air

Just try to be mad when this diffuser recipe is running. These essential oils can calm even the angriest of beasts. The oils and their properties include antidepressant, nervine, sedative, aphrodisiac, and tonic components.

Yield: 1 application

Recipe

2 drops grapefruit oil

2 drops patchouli oil

2 drops lavender oil

Water

Follow your directions for using essential oils in your particular brand of diffuser. Ensure that your diffuser does not use heat but runs by vibration, sound waves, or another cold-steam type of process. Choose the essential oils needed for your condition, then add water and oils to the diffuser. Run your diffuser as needed to permeate the air with therapeutic properties and achieve the results you desire.

Happy Rubdown

These oils contain sedative, aphrodisiac, tonic, antidepressant, and calming properties that help to reduce the stress and replace it with peaceful feelings of zen.

Yield: ½ ounce

Recipe

1 drop lavender oil

1 drop clary sage oil

1 drop sandalwood oil
½ ounce carrier oil

Pour the essential oils, carrier oil, and any remaining ingredients into a small glass container, bowl, or jar. Swirl or whisk to mix the ingredients and apply lightly to the area desired. Keep essential oil mixture away from open wounds, mucus membranes, genitals, eyes, and sensitive areas. Repeat application as needed, usually 2–3 times daily. You may cover area with linen or cloth to protect clothing and furniture. Store unused portion in a glass jar or container with a tight-fitting lid in a cool, dark area for up to 3 months.

Breathe In My Joy

Breathe in this delightful aroma while chanting the phrase, "My life is good; my life is good." Anger can get the best of any of us at some point during any day. Inhaling essential oils can reduce the adrenaline coursing through our veins and bring a sense of calm and peace to us. Replace those negative, anger-filled vibes with healthy, positive feelings. The properties contained in these essential oils include antidepressant, euphoric, aphrodisiac, tonic, and nervine compounds.

Yield: 1 application

RECIPE
1 drop clary sage oil
1 drop lavender oil

Choose your essential oil and apply to the palm of your hand, an oil inhaler, or a tissue. Bring the essential oils close to your nostrils and inhale the aroma deeply. You can cover one nostril at a time with your thumb and, if you prefer, alternate nostrils. This process sends the properties straight to your brain and the effects are immediate. You can complete this process 3–4 times daily.

Bathe in Euphoria

Just let all that small stuff go while relaxing in this pleasant, aromatic wonderland. These essential oils are reputed to calm the nerves, assuage anger, and bring peace and hope to him or her with their sedative, cephalic, tonic, and nervine properties.

Yield: 1 application

RECIPE

3 drops grapefruit oil

3 drops spearmint oil

2 drops lavender oil

1 drop bergamot oil

1 tablespoon carrier oil

1 tablespoon milk (optional for adults, recommended for children)

As you begin to fill the tub with water, pour the chosen essential oils and carrier oil into the running water. Run a warm, not hot, bath. Water that is too hot will cause the essential oils to dissipate. You may add 1 tablespoon of milk to the water; this ensures that the essential oils will not stick to your skin, but will mix with the water. You may soak in the water as long as you are comfortable. Dry your feet well once you get out of the water, as the oils will cause them to be slippery, increasing your chances of falling. Rinse the tub of any remaining oils.

Massage that Madness

So how can anyone stay mad while receiving a massage? Throw in these essential oils and it becomes impossible to have an angry bone in your body. Just relax and go with it while receiving the properties such as aphrodisiac, antidepressant, nervine, and sedative compounds.

Yield: 2 fluid ounces

RECIPE

2 drops lavender oil

2 drops patchouli oil

2 drops ylang-ylang oil

1 drop clary sage oil

2 fluid ounces carrier oil

Pour the essential oils and the carrier oil into a small glass container, bowl, or jar. Swirl to mix the ingredients and use to lightly massage the area desired. Keep essential oil mixture away from open wounds, mucus membranes, genitals, eyes, and sensitive areas. Repeat application as needed. Store unused portion in a glass jar or container with a tight-fitting lid in a cool, dark area for up to 3 months.

Keeping it Real Bath Salts

I know that anger can get the best of me sometimes. When I can't let it go, this is the blend I turn to. It gives me the ability to focus on the good intentions of others and to not dwell on the haters. Om … The therapeutic properties in this recipe contain such soul-healing compounds as aphrodisiac, sedative, nervine, tonic, antidepressant, and calming agents.

Yield: 3 cups

RECIPE
5 drops vetiver oil
5 drops ylang-ylang oil
5 drops myrrh oil
2 tablespoons carrier oil
3 cups salts
1 tablespoon milk (optional for adults, recommended for children)

Use any type of salt you prefer: pink Himalayan salt, sea salt, Epsom salts, etc. In a small container, add the essential oils to the desired type of salt. Stir until well blended. Screw lid onto container tightly. Leave mixture in a dark area for 24 hours and then stir mixture again. Run the bathwater. Once the tub is full of water, you can add the milk, and then add ½ cup of the bath salt mixture to bathwater as you get into the tub. You may stay in the tub as long as the temperature is comfortable. Dry your feet well when you get out of the bath, as the oils are slippery and can cause you to fall. Store remainder in a glass jar or container with a tight-fitting lid in a cool, dark area for up to 3 months. These jars make attractive, inexpensive, and healing gifts!

Anxiety

Anxiety is a feeling caused by stress, fear, or it can be from an unknown cause. A person with anxiety often worries, feels afraid, and cannot cope normally in a calm or relaxed manner. Essential oils can help to alleviate fears and worries and bring a person peace, calm, and joy. People with too much of the vata dosha are often plagued with unnecessary anxiety.

Essential Oils

Basil, chamomile, clary sage, cypress, frankincense, geranium, hyssop, jasmine, juniper, lavender, lemon, marjoram, melissa, neroli, orange, peppermint, petitgrain, rose, sandalwood, and ylang-ylang

Fearless Oil

This is a massage oil to use for those times you are very worried and anxious about the outside world. Everything just seems to drop away while you melt into a peaceful, dreamy state of relaxation. I like to use this when I am going to have a party or some company and I know it's going to be fun, but I just have stress and anxiety about trivial concerns. I use this massage blend on my chest and neck and will soon feel relaxed, happy, and calm in just minutes and am then assured that I am present enough to help others feel more at ease. This blend works well due to its nervine and antidepressant properties.

Yield: 1 fluid ounce

RECIPE
2 drops lavender oil
2 drops marjoram oil
2 drops jasmine oil
4 drops vitamin E oil
1 fluid ounce carrier oil

Pour the essential oils and the carrier oil into a small glass container, bowl, or jar. Swirl to mix the ingredients and use to massage lightly the area desired, such as neck, chest, back, temples, or soles of feet. Keep essential oil mixture away from open wounds, mucus membranes, genitals, eyes, and sensitive areas. Repeat application as needed. Store unused portion in a glass jar or container with a tight-fitting lid in a cool, dark area for up to 3 months.

Bathing Release

Take control of your thoughts and emotions as you revel in this comforting bath time retreat. These essential oils are reputed to help you ease your anxious mind. Antianxiety, antidepressant, and tonic properties make this recipe perfect for those anxiety-provoking days that lead to sleepless, anxious nights.

Yield: 1 application

RECIPE
6 drops frankincense oil
5 drops neroli oil
2 drops ylang-ylang oil
1 tablespoon carrier oil
1 tablespoon milk (optional for adults, recommended for children)

As you begin to fill the tub with water, pour the chosen essential oils and carrier oil into the running water. Run a warm, not hot, bath. Water that is too hot will cause the essential oils to dissipate. You may add 1 tablespoon of milk to the water; this ensures that the essential oils will not stick to your skin, but will mix with the water. You may soak in the water as long as you are comfortable. Dry your feet well once you get out of the water, as the oils will cause them to be slippery, increasing your chances of falling. Rinse the tub of any remaining oils.

Power Up

This rub has been reputed to whisk away your fears and fill you with the power you need to confront the issues at hand. These essential oils are perfect for empowerment and determination and letting all those worries drift away. Find support in the antidepressant and stimulating properties inherent in these oils.

Yield: ½ ounce

RECIPE
2 drops orange oil
2 drops jasmine oil
2 drops cypress oil
3 drops vitamin E oil
½ ounce carrier oil

Pour the essential oils, carrier oil, and any remaining ingredients into a small glass container, bowl, or jar. Swirl or whisk to mix the ingredients and apply lightly to the area desired. Keep essential oil mixture away from open wounds, mucus membranes, genitals, eyes, and sensitive areas. Repeat application as needed, usually 2–3 times daily. You may cover area with linen or cloth to protect clothing and furniture. Store unused portion in a glass jar or container with a tight-fitting lid in a cool, dark area for up to 3 months.

No Fear Inhale

This aroma will provide a quick boost of confidence when going for a job interview or other anxiety-provoking situation. Calming and sedative therapeutic properties work to ease your fears, thereby enabling you to think clearly and precisely. Help to take control of your fears and worries by breathing in this powerful blend.

Yield: 1 application

RECIPE
1 drop frankincense oil
1 drop lavender oil

Choose your essential oil and apply to the palm of your hand, an oil inhaler, or a tissue. Bring the essential oils close to your nostrils and inhale the aroma deeply. You can cover one nostril at a time with your thumb and, if you prefer, alternate nostrils. This process sends the properties straight to your brain and the effects are immediate. You can complete this process 3–4 times daily.

No Anxiety Sugar Scrub

These oils work well together to reduce anxiety and bring a sense of calm. This scrub will not only provide you with the therapeutic properties of the oils, but will also make your skin soft and smelling beautiful.

Yield: 8 ounces

RECIPE

8 ounces sugar (white or turbinado)

1 fluid ounce coconut oil

1 fluid ounce vegetable glycerin

1 fluid ounce liquid castile soap

½ teaspoon vitamin E oil

10 drops jasmine oil

10 drops juniper oil

10 drops melissa oil

10 drops rose oil

10 drops neroli oil

Combine ingredients without mashing too much. Spread paste onto skin or area desired and rub in lightly. Do not apply to genitals, eyes, sensitive areas, or mucus membranes. Sugar scrub should never be applied to the face. Let set for 1 minute, and then gently rise off. Keep in a glass jar with a tight-fitting lid in a cool, dark area for up to 1 month.

Calm

When the stress of our daily lives gets to be a little too much, we often look outside of ourselves for something bigger to bring calmness, peace, and tranquility to our soul. Using essential oils for this purpose can be very effective. Experiment with essential oils to find the one that works best for you. Doing activities like meditation, prayer, or taking a walk can calm you and bring about grounding in stressful situations. People often feel stress, worry, and get anxious for an unknown reason. A diffuser with particular essential oils added to it can be enormously calming, so I naturally run one every day of my life. Using essential oils can greatly reduce the worry and stress that is keeping your calm at bay.

Essential Oils

Bergamot, clary sage, geranium, jasmine, lavender, mandarin, neroli, vetiver, and ylang-ylang

Calm Me Linen Powder

If you are having anxious nights, sprinkle some of this under your sheets to bring a sense of calm to you while you sleep. These aromas impart an aura of peace and contentment as you drift off into slumber. The therapeutic properties contained in these essential oils include sedative, antidepressant, and nervine components.

Yield: ¼ cup

RECIPE
3 drops vetiver oil
3 drops clary sage oil
3 drops ylang-ylang oil
¼ cup cornstarch
4 drops vitamin E oil

Place the ingredients into a mason jar, stirring well with a whisk. Carefully poke holes into the lid, use this as a shaker, and shake the ingredients into pillowcases or under sheet areas as needed. You can get a piece of plastic wrap and place it over the jar and under the lid to keep powder from spilling out when not in use. Store in a glass jar or container with a tight-fitting lid in a cool, dark, and dry area for up to 3 months.

Calming Spray

When you are getting scattered in your actions or feeling as if your mind and thoughts are over loaded, spray this everywhere to help you calm down and think things through more rationally. When feeling overwhelmed with emotions, try to bring yourself into a more peaceful and understanding state of mind by using this recipe. These oils can help bring calm with their tranquilizing, antidepressant, sedative, and hypotensive properties.

Yield: 2 fluid ounces

RECIPE
10 drops vetiver oil
10 drops mandarin essential oil
4 drops vitamin E oil
2 fluid ounces water

Add all ingredients to a dark-colored spray bottle. Check for material steadfastness before spraying on fabric. Shake the bottle and spray onto area desired. Do not spray into or on open wounds, genitals, eyes, or mucus membranes. Store in a cool, dark area for up to 3 months. Shake well before each use to combine the ingredients.

Bring It Down Bath
When you feel like you are losing control of your emotions, use this bath recipe to restore order in your mind and soul. Take this bath and come out feeling rejuvenated, rested, and calm. Essential oils can change the course of your brain receptors with their sedative and antidepressant properties.

Yield: 1 application

RECIPE
8 drops jasmine oil
4 drops lavender oil
1 tablespoon carrier oil
1 tablespoon milk (optional for adults, recommended for children)

As you begin to fill the tub with water, pour the chosen essential oils and carrier oil into the running water. Run a warm, not hot, bath. Water that is too hot will cause the essential oils to dissipate. You may add 1 tablespoon of milk to the water; this ensures that the essential oils will not stick to your skin, but will mix with the water. You may soak in the water as long as you are comfortable. Dry your feet well once you get out of the water, as the oils will cause them to be slippery, increasing your chances of falling. Rinse the tub of any remaining oils.

Calming Massage Blend

Sometimes we just need a little bit of help in coping with the demands we are unceasingly confronted with. Couple these essential oils with your massage and it will help you to be in a calm, relaxed state of mind for the rest of the day. The powerful calming agents are nervine, sedative, and tranquilizing components to bring you to a meditative state where all is right with the world.

Yield: 1 fluid ounce

RECIPE
4 drops neroli oil
4 drops bergamot oil
8 drops lavender oil
3 drops vitamin E oil
1 fluid ounce carrier oil

Pour the essential oils and the carrier oil into a small glass container, bowl, or jar. Swirl to mix the ingredients and use to massage lightly the area desired, such as temples, neck, chest, back, or soles of feet. Keep essential oil mixture away from open wounds, mucus membranes, genitals, eyes, and sensitive areas. Repeat application as needed. Store unused portion in a glass jar or container with a tight-fitting lid in a cool, dark area for up to 3 months.

Peaceful Air Diffuser

This recipe is great for calming someone down that lives in your household or that you work with. You can run this diffuser in a negative environment and boost the peaceful atmosphere that you desire. The sedative and antidepressant therapeutic properties of this blend will calm and relax even the most uptight person.

Yield: 1 application

RECIPE

2 drops vetiver oil

3 drops geranium oil

Water

Follow your directions for using essential oils in your particular brand of diffuser. Ensure that your diffuser does not use heat but runs by vibration, sound waves, or another cold-steam type of process. Choose the essential oils needed for your condition, then add water and oils to the diffuser. Run your diffuser as needed to permeate the air with therapeutic properties and achieve the results you desire.

Chill Out Bath Salts

Overextending yourself and multitasking often leaves you with the inability to calm down before bed. Apply these calming salts to your bath and you will come out thinking only about sleep … not the million things you have to do tomorrow. The sleep-inducing properties of this recipe are its sedative, antidepressant, and tranquilizing agents.

Yield: 3 cups

RECIPE

5 drops vetiver oil

5 drops clary sage oil

5 drops lavender oil

2 tablespoons carrier oil

3 cups salts

1 tablespoon milk (optional for adults, recommended for children)

Use any type of salt you prefer: pink Himalayan salt, sea salt, Epsom salts, Etc. Add essential oils and carrier oil to salt and Stir until well blended. Screw lid onto container tightly. Leave mixture in a dark area for 24 hours and then stir mixture again. Run the bathwater. Once the tub is full of water, you can add the milk, and then add ½ cup of the bath salt mixture to bathwater as you get into the tub. These jars make attractive, inexpensive, and healing gifts! You may add a tablespoon of milk to the bathwater to prevent the oils from adhering to your skin. Store remainder in a glass jar or container with a tight-fitting lid in a cool, dark area for up to 3 months.

Desperation

Desperation is an all-consuming emotion that fills one with angst, sadness, hopelessness, worry, anxiety, fear, and a need to meet a particular outcome through any means possible. Balancing your emotions and thinking with a clear, level head is what you should strive for in any desperate situation. These recipes will help you to make plans to change the situation and take control. These essential oils promote clear-headedness, focus, and clarity.

Essential Oils

Black pepper, cassia, cedarwood, clary sage, dill, geranium, jasmine, lavender, lemon, Palo Santo, patchouli, sandalwood, and ylang-ylang

Instant Inhale

To bring yourself back to earth quickly and counteract your feelings of desperation, inhale this aroma and feel yourself start to calm down immediately. When I am desperate to find a solution, and to be a part of the solution, I turn to these oils to open my consciousness and begin outlining steps to problem-solve.

Yield: 1 application

RECIPE
1 drop melissa oil

or

1 drop lavender oil

or

1 drop sandalwood oil

Choose your essential oil and apply to the palm of your hand, an oil inhaler, or a tissue. Bring the essential oils close to your nostrils and inhale the aroma deeply. You can cover one nostril at a time with your thumb and, if you prefer, alternate nostrils. This process sends the properties straight to your brain and the effects are immediate. You can complete this process 3–4 times daily.

Grounding Foot Rub

The soles of the feet transport essential oils to every cell in your body in a matter of minutes. These essential oils will help you to feel grounded very quickly. When you feel your thoughts going every which way and you can't seem to focus on the important matter at hand, this is the blend for you. Corral those desperate thoughts and bring a solution to the table by applying this recipe, soaking up the properties that will help you to be grounded and focused.

Yield: 1 application

RECIPE
1 drop clary sage
1 drop geranium oil
1 drop cedarwood oil
3 drops vitamin E oil
½ teaspoon carrier oil

Pour the essential oils, carrier oil, and any remaining ingredients into a small glass container, bowl, or jar. Swirl or whisk to mix the ingredients and apply lightly to the area desired, such as pressure points, neck, soles of feet, temples, or chest. Keep essential oil mixture away from open wounds, mucus membranes, genitals, eyes, and sensitive areas. Repeat application as needed, usually 2–3 times daily. You may cover area with linen or cloth to protect clothing and furniture. Store unused portion in a glass jar or container with a tight-fitting lid in a cool, dark area for up to 3 months.

Balance Bath and Shower Bomb

Desperation can have you falling into a depression and feeling like you have nowhere to turn or drive you into a panic-fueled mess where you only make bad decisions. These oils will work together to balance your thoughts and assist your mind in grasping the positive aspects of your life, coming up with a solution to your problem, and putting that desperation behind you. These bath and shower bombs are said to infuse your bath with hope-lifting, problem-solving, fear-quenching oils.

Yield: 8–12 bombs

RECIPE
1 cup baking soda
½ cup citric acid
½ cup cornstarch
½ cup Epsom salts, fine grained
15 drops lavender oil
15 drops patchouli oil
10 drops jasmine oil
½ teaspoon carrier oil
¾ teaspoon water
spray bottle (water)

In a large bowl, mix your dry ingredients together until fine with a whisk. In a tiny jar with a lid, add your wet ingredients and shake to mix. You may add a couple drops of food coloring to the wet jar. Extremely slowly, add the wet ingredients to the dry ingredients while whisking rapidly. If fizzing takes place, whisk until it is mixed. Once the ingredients are well mixed, it should be the texture of slightly damp sand. Add a spray or two of water if needed. Once the mixture is the consistency you like, form into balls; I just smash mine down into ice cube trays or muffin tins. You can use cute molds, but you must work rapidly as mixture will dry out quickly. Leave in open air, uncovered, in a room where they will not be disturbed for 12–24 hours. Once they are dry, you can place 1–2 bombs into your bath or directly into the spray of the shower and they will fizz and release their aromatic and healing properties. Store unused portion in an airtight container for up to 6 months.

Salve of Hope

This recipe contains essential oils that have been reported to bring hope, peace, and calm to those suffering from desperation.

Yield: 1 tablespoon

RECIPE

7 drops Palo Santo oil

5 drops lavender oil

3 drops ylang-ylang oil

1 teaspoon beeswax pellets

4 drops vitamin E oil

3 teaspoons carrier oil

Heat the beeswax and the carrier oil in a glass bowl in the microwave for 1 ½–2 minutes, until just melted, or on low on the stovetop. If you open the door every 15 seconds, you can avoid the popping of the wax and oil and overheating. Carefully remove the container from the microwave and stir. Drip a drop of the melted oil and wax onto the counter, after 1 minute check for consistency. If it is too thin, add more beeswax to the container; if it is too thick, add more carrier oil. Add the vitamin E oil and the essential oil to the heated mixture in the container. Whisk lightly, and it will begin hardening immediately. Pour into containers. Ensure your containers are glass or tin to prevent leeching of chemicals. Once cool, apply to wrists, temples, neck, or soles of feet. Do not apply to mucus membranes, eyes, genitals, or open wounds. Label containers and store in a dark, dry area for up to 1 year.

Exhaustion

Exhaustion is usually caused by physical overexertion, but it's sometimes caused by mental fatigue as well. A person can oftentimes rid himself or herself of exhaustion by simply sleeping an adequate amount of time. Exhaustion can sometimes cause a person to be hospitalized if dehydration, mental exhaustion, or a number of other factors are also present. Caregivers and civil servants are a couple of examples of professions that are prone to exhaustion due to constant demand on their time, patience, energy, and peace of mind. These recipes have the restorative powers to revitalize your energy and return you to that peaceful frame of mind.

Essential Oils

Bergamot, basil, cassia, cinnamon, citrus, lavender, lemon, lime, eucalyptus, frankincense, grapefruit, peppermint, rosemary, wild orange, and white fir

Give Me Strength Bath Salts

When you are not feeling your best but still have a long day to get through, this bath will revive and energize you to face the day ahead. These particular essential oils are thought to give you strength, endurance, and energy with their antidepressant and restorative properties. Most salts contain powerful minerals in their own right and will impart healthy benefits to your body. Eliminate that mental and physical exhaustion by immersing yourself in this wonderfully energizing salt bath.

Yield: 3 cups

RECIPE
7 drops bergamot oil
7 drops wild orange oil
7 drops lime oil
2 tablespoons carrier oil
5 drops vitamin E oil
3 cups salts
1 tablespoon milk (optional for adults, recommended for children)

Use any type of salt you prefer: pink Himalayan salt, sea salt, Epsom salts, etc. In a small container, add the essential oils to the desired type of salt. Stir until well blended. Screw lid onto container tightly. Leave mixture in a dark area for 24 hours and then stir mixture again. Run the bathwater. Once the tub is full of water, you can add the milk, and then add ½ cup of the bath salt mixture to bathwater as you get into the tub. You may stay in the tub as long as the temperature is comfortable. Dry your feet well when you get out of the bath, as the oils are slippery and can cause you to fall. Store remainder in a glass jar or container with a tight-fitting lid in a cool, dark area for up to 3 months. These jars make attractive, inexpensive, and healing gifts!

I Need Energy Inhale

This inhale is a great afternoon pick-me-up that only takes a couple of seconds to complete. Carry a vial of either of these oils in your car or purse and smell them when you start getting weary and feel that exhaustion setting in. The energy-boosting and tonic properties in these oils will clear your head and give you the strength to make it through the rest of the day.

Yield: 1 application

RECIPE

1 drop bergamot oil

or

1 drop peppermint oil

Choose your essential oil and apply to the palm of your hand, an oil inhaler, or a tissue. Bring the essential oils close to your nostrils and inhale the aroma deeply. You can cover one nostril at a time with your thumb and, if you prefer, alternate nostrils. This process sends the properties straight to your brain and the effects are immediate. You can complete this process 3–4 times daily.

Energy Bath and Shower Bombs

These oils have the power to get you going and keep you going all day. Just put one of these bombs in your bath or shower and absorb the energizing therapeutic properties that inundate the water and air. They can infuse your mind, body, and spirit with energetic impulses.

Yield: 12–18 balls

RECIPE

1 cup baking soda

½ cup citric acid

½ cup cornstarch

½ cup Epsom salts, fine grained

15 drops white fir oil

15 drops frankincense oil

½ teaspoon carrier oil
¾ teaspoon water
spray bottle (water)

In a large bowl, mix your dry ingredients together until fine with a whisk. In a tiny jar with a lid, add your wet ingredients and shake to mix. You may add a couple drops of food coloring to the wet jar. Extremely slowly, add the wet ingredients to the dry ingredients while whisking rapidly. If fizzing takes place, whisk until it is mixed. Once the ingredients are well mixed, it should be the texture of slightly damp sand. Add a spray or two of water if needed. Once the mixture is the consistency you like, form into balls; I just smash mine down into ice cube trays or muffin tins. You can use cute molds, but you must work rapidly as mixture will dry out quickly. Leave in open air, uncovered, in a room where they will not be disturbed for 12–24 hours. Once they are dry, you can place 1–2 bombs into your bath or directly into the spray of the shower and they will fizz and release their aromatic and healing properties. Store unused portion in an airtight container for up to 6 months.

Fear

In certain situations, fear is a healthy response to outside stimuli. In other cases, it is unwarranted and causes an overtaxing reaction in our nervous systems. Fear can come from many sources: environment, social situations, unbalanced doshas, mentality, or from anxiety about events, certain or uncertain. To keep fear at bay, we can use essential oils to promote feelings of well-being.

Essential Oils
Bergamot, chamomile, clary sage, fennel, frankincense, geranium, grapefruit, jasmine, lavender, marjoram, neroli, orange, sandalwood, vetiver, and ylang-ylang

Overcoming Fear Powder
Kids love this powder, especially if they are prone to nightmares. Sprinkle under the sheets for a peaceful night's sleep. Kids can sprinkle it themselves and take power over

their fear. (Use only with children over the age of four years.) I use this often when I know I am going to toss and turn all night with worry or anxiety. The essential oils in this blend contain antidepressant and sedative properties to calm that overactive mind.

Yield: ¼ cup

RECIPE
3 drops orange oil
3 drops neroli oil
3 drops chamomile oil
¼ cup cornstarch
4 drops vitamin E oil

Place the ingredients into a mason jar, stirring well with a whisk. Carefully poke holes into the lid, use this as a shaker, and shake the ingredients into pillowcases or under sheet areas as needed. You can get a piece of plastic wrap and place it over the jar and under the lid to keep powder from spilling out when not in use. Store in a glass jar or container with a tight-fitting lid in a cool, dark, and dry area for up to 3 months.

Monster Zapper Spray

This is the concoction many children (over s old) are raised with. They can keep it by their beds and wipe out any monsters that approach during the night. The sedative and antidepressant properties in this blend help to dispel fear and negative feelings and assist in getting a good night's sleep. It works wonderfully, and they aren't even aware that sedative and tranquilizing properties are working hard to get them to sleep without fear.

Yield: 2 fluid ounces

RECIPE
10 drops orange oil
8 drops lavender oil
5 drops grapefruit oil
3 drops vitamin E oil

1 tablespoon witch hazel

2 fluid ounces water

Add all ingredients to a dark-colored spray bottle. Check for material steadfastness before spraying on fabric. Shake the bottle and spray onto area desired, such as body, hair, home, car, or office. Do not spray into or on open wounds, genitals, eyes, or mucus membranes. Store in a cool, dark area for up to 3 months. (My grandchildren stored theirs on their bookcases next to their beds.) Shake well before each use to combine the ingredients.

Protection Spray

I love to spray this around my home if someone negative has been present or if I have received bad news and am fearful of the future. These essential oils are reported to bring protection and peace to those who use it. This blend is fortified with tranquilizing and sedative properties to dispel any fears you may have.

Yield: 2 fluid ounces

RECIPE

15 drops neroli oil

5 drops chamomile oil

5 drops vetiver oil

1 tablespoon witch hazel

2 fluid ounces water

Add all ingredients to a dark-colored spray bottle. Check for material steadfastness before spraying on fabric. Shake the bottle and spray onto area desired, such as body, hair, home, car, or office. Do not spray into or on open wounds, genitals, eyes, or mucus membranes. Store in a cool, dark area for up to 3 months. Shake well before each use to combine the ingredients.

Fear Be Gone Bath

Sometimes in life we are consumed by fears—some of them warranted, some of them imagined. This bath will help us put things into perspective and decide the course of action that needs to be taken. The sedative and tranquilizing properties in this blend work together to promote positive sleep and dreams.

Yield: 1 application

RECIPE

6 drops lavender oil

4 drops vetiver oil

4 drops frankincense oil

3 drops orange oil

5 drops clary sage oil

1 tablespoon carrier oil

1 tablespoon milk (optional for adults, recommended for children)

As you begin to fill the tub with water, pour the chosen essential oils and carrier oil into the running water. Run a warm, not hot, bath. Water that is too hot will cause the essential oils to dissipate. You may add 1 tablespoon of milk to the water; this ensures that the essential oils will not stick to your skin, but will mix with the water. You may soak in the water as long as you are comfortable. Dry your feet well once you get out of the water, as the oils will cause them to be slippery, increasing your chances of falling. Rinse the tub of any remaining oils.

Fear Dispelling Diffuser

Run this diffuser recipe to keep fears at bay and to increase the power that resides inside of you. These essential oils promote strength and courage with their aphrodisiacal, euphoric, and sedative properties. I like to run this diffuser at work or at home if I know a conflict is brewing and I need to take charge and not be a nervous or timid wreck. This blend gives me the ability to be strong!

Yield: 1 application

RECIPE

4 drops vetiver oil

5 drops clary sage oil

3 drops ylang-ylang oil
Water

Follow your directions for using essential oils in your particular brand of diffuser. Ensure that your diffuser does not use heat but runs by vibration, sound waves, or another cold-steam type of process. Choose the essential oils needed for your condition, then add water and oils to the diffuser. Run your diffuser as needed to permeate the air with therapeutic properties and achieve the results you desire.

Evaporating Fear Massage

The essential oils in this massage recipe are reputed to give you courage and to quell anxiety. The therapeutic properties of this blend include tranquilizing, sedative, and aphrodisiac elements.

Yield: 1 fluid ounce

RECIPE
3 drops lavender oil
3 drops vetiver oil
3 drops chamomile oil
3 drops vitamin E oil
1 fluid ounce carrier oil

Pour the essential oils and the carrier oil into a small glass container, bowl, or jar. Swirl to mix the ingredients and use to massage lightly the area desired, such as temples, neck, chest, back, or soles of feet. Keep essential oil mixture away from open wounds, mucus membranes, genitals, eyes, and sensitive areas. Repeat application as needed. Store unused portion in a glass jar or container with a tight-fitting lid in a cool, dark area for up to 3 months.

Take a Stand Bath Salts

This recipe is full of properties such as antidepressant, sedative, and tonic components to help dispel any negative emotions and replace them with positive thoughts and feelings. Eliminate fear with the inner strength-inducing essential oils of this recipe.

Yield: 3 cups

RECIPE

7 drops neroli oil

7 drops fennel oil

7 drops sandalwood oil

2 tablespoons carrier oil

5 drops vitamin E oil

3 cups salts

1 tablespoon milk (optional for adults, recommended for children)

Use any type of salt you prefer: pink Himalayan salt, sea salt, Epsom salts, etc. In a small container, add the essential oils to the desired type of salt. Stir until well blended. Screw lid onto container tightly. Leave mixture in a dark area for 24 hours and then stir mixture again. Run the bathwater. Once the tub is full of water, you can add the milk, and then add ½ cup of the bath salt mixture to bathwater as you get into the tub. You may stay in the tub as long as the temperature is comfortable. Dry your feet well when you get out of the bath, as the oils are slippery and can cause you to fall. Store remainder in a glass jar or container with a tight-fitting lid in a cool, dark area for up to 3 months. These jars make attractive, inexpensive, and healing gifts!

Gloom

Gloom casts a shadow over everyone even if only one person is suffering from it. These essential oils bring about positive emotions and peace to a gloomy, downtrodden atmosphere. The essential oils in these recipes have been used forever to help people overcome that gloomy disposition and replace it with light and love.

Essential Oils

Palo Santo, marjoram, rosemary, neroli, sage, mandarin, bay laurel, bergamot, ginseng, cinnamon, geranium, rose, and sandalwood

Laughter in the Air Diffuser

These mood-enhancing essential oils can banish the gloom from any room. Try this the next time you or someone else is holding on to those negative thoughts. Run this diffuser to lighten the mood and bring a little happiness into your life.

Yield: 1 application

RECIPE
5 drops bergamot oil
5 drops bay laurel oil
5 drops neroli oil
Water

Follow your directions for using essential oils in your particular brand of diffuser. Ensure that your diffuser does not use heat but runs by vibration, sound waves, or another cold-steam type of process. Choose the essential oils needed for your condition, then add water and oils to the diffuser. Run your diffuser as needed to permeate the air with therapeutic properties and achieve the results you desire.

Gloom Dispelling Sugar Scrub

When feeling like you are trapped in gloom, use this sugar scrub to lift your spirits. These essential oils are known for their joyful and energizing therapeutic properties.

Yield: 8 ounces

RECIPE
8 ounces sugar (white or turbinado)
1 fluid ounce coconut oil
1 fluid ounce vegetable glycerin
1 fluid ounce liquid castile soap
½ teaspoon vitamin E oil
10 drops Palo Santo oil

10 drops neroli oil

10 drops bergamot oil

10 drops bay laurel oil

10 drops geranium oil

Combine ingredients without mashing too much. Spread paste onto skin or area desired and rub in lightly. Do not apply to genitals, eyes, sensitive areas, or mucus membranes. Sugar scrub should never be applied to the face. Let set for 1 minute, and then gently rise off. Keep in a glass jar with a tight-fitting lid in a cool, dark area for up to 1 month.

Joy

Pure, unadulterated joy is an elusive emotion that we all want and strive to achieve. I personally find joy in a simple collusion with nature. We work daily to bring joy into our lives and into the lives of our families. These essential oils are reported throughout the world to help people to achieve this feeling of bliss. The list of essential oils below is full of joy- and happiness-inducing properties.

Essential Oils

Bergamot, coriander, geranium, grapefruit, jasmine, lime, neroli, orange, palmarosa, Roman chamomile, rose, sandalwood, spearmint, tangerine, and ylang-ylang

Jumping for Joy Massage Oil

This massage oil has the greatest blend of essential oils in it that are full of joy-producing therapeutic properties. Let yourself be immersed into a world of euphoria and happiness while this recipe is being applied. In this recipe, the vitamin E oil not only works wonders for your skin, but acts as a preservative, allowing you to store your massage oil for future usage.

Yield: 1 fluid ounce

Recipe

5 drops jasmine oil

5 drops palmarosa oil

5 drops tangerine oil

5 drops ylang-ylang oil

1 fluid ounce carrier oil

3 drops vitamin E oil

Pour the essential oils and the carrier oil into a small glass container, bowl, or jar. Swirl to mix the ingredients and use to massage lightly the area desired, such as temples, neck, chest, back, or soles of feet. Keep essential oil mixture away from open wounds, mucus membranes, genitals, eyes, and sensitive areas. Repeat application as needed. Store unused portion in a glass jar or container with a tight-fitting lid in a cool, dark area for up to 3 months.

Joyous Spray

When you want a pick-me-up, or want to increase your happiness, this is the recipe you can turn to. These essential oils have been used throughout history to bring joy to gatherings of people and during holidays. Spray it everywhere; this blend will fill the space with joy and also impart a delightful aroma to any room.

Yield: 2 fluid ounces

RECIPE

9 drops rose oil

7 drops orange oil

5 drops lemon oil

4 drops Roman chamomile oil

2 fluid ounces water

4 drops vitamin E oil

Add all ingredients to a dark-colored spray bottle. Check for material steadfastness before spraying on fabric. Shake the bottle and spray onto area desired, such as body, hair, home, car, or office. Do not spray into or on open wounds, genitals, eyes, or mucus membranes. Store in a cool, dark area for up to 3 months. Shake well before each use to combine the ingredients.

Joyful Holiday Air

Every time I smell this, I can't help but think of the winter celebrations that take place each year. These oils are diffused throughout our family's homes during the holidays and the aroma just gets us in a celebratory mood and fills us with joy. Just smelling this scent helps me to be happier and excited for what the days ahead are bringing. The invigorating properties in this blend smell as wonderful as they work.

Yield: 1 application

RECIPE
8 drops spearmint oil
3 drops lime oil
3 drops orange oil
1 drop grapefruit oil
Water

Follow your directions for using essential oils in your particular brand of diffuser. Ensure that your diffuser does not use heat but runs by vibration, sound waves, or another cold-steam type of process. Choose the essential oils needed for your condition, then add water and oils to the diffuser. Run your diffuser as needed to permeate the air with therapeutic properties and achieve the results you desire.

Joyful Lip Balm

This lip balm has the therapeutic properties needed to stimulate those parts of our brains responsible for happiness. Wear this when you are feeling a little down for a quick lift of your spirits.

Yield: 1 tablespoon

RECIPE
3 teaspoons grape seed oil
½ teaspoon beeswax pellets
4 drops vitamin E oil
3 drops bergamot oil
3 drops pink tangerine oil

Melt the beeswax and the carrier oil in a glass bowl in the microwave until most of the beeswax is melted. You can also use a pan on the stovetop on low. Cool slightly. Add the vitamin E and the essential oils and stir or whisk quickly. With a spoon, drip a drop of the mixture onto the counter and Let set for 1 minute. Pull your finger through the drop and check for consistency. If mixture is too thin, add more beeswax; if it is too thick, add more oil. Once desired consistency is acquired, immediately pour into small balm container (glass or metal) with a lid. After mixture cools, cover and store in a cool, dark area for up to 6 months.

Misery

Misery is one of the worst emotions to deal with. Misery invokes heartache, heartbreak, grief, loneliness, overall sadness, and despair in everyone associated with a person overcome by misery; everyone is affected, not just the person who is suffering. Plants have been used for thousands of years as a coping mechanism to deal with misery. We are lucky today that we don't have to wait for these plants to bloom, we have a high-quality concentration in the form of essential oil at our disposal every day. These essential oils are full of therapeutic properties that can help to bring our misery to an end and fill our hearts with hope, positivity, and contentment.

Essential Oils

Bergamot, cinnamon, clove, frankincense, ginger, helichrysum, jasmine, lemon, mandarin, neroli, orange, palmarosa, petitgrain, rose, rosewood, and ylang-ylang

Favorite Spray

This spray is one of the most positive, uplifting, and mood-enhancing aromas available. Try this recipe in your home to banish any misery and bring joy to your household.

Yield: 2 fluid ounces

RECIPE
7 drops melissa oil
3 drops ylang-ylang oil

3 drops rosewood oil

3 drops petitgrain oil

1 tablespoon witch hazel

2 fluid ounces water

Add all ingredients to a dark-colored spray bottle. Check for material steadfastness before spraying on fabric. Shake the bottle and spray onto area desired, such as body, hair, home, car, or office. Do not spray into or on open wounds, genitals, eyes, or mucus membranes. Store in a cool, dark area for up to 3 months. Shake well before each use to combine the ingredients.

Bliss in a Jar Sugar Scrub

Use this recipe before your bath or shower. Immersing in these healing and mood-uplifting essential oils will bring a joy of the spirit to everyone who smells this delightful blend. The invigorating scrubbing action coupled with the healing oils will help you to feel invigorated and joyful.

Yield: 8 ounces

RECIPE

8 ounces sugar (white or turbinado)

1 fluid ounce coconut oil

1 fluid ounce vegetable glycerin

1 fluid ounce liquid castile soap

½ teaspoon vitamin E oil

10 drops orange oil

10 drops lemon oil

10 drops melissa oil

10 drops frankincense oil

10 drops geranium oil

Combine ingredients without mashing too much. Spread paste onto skin or area desired and rub in lightly. Do not apply to genitals, eyes, sensitive areas, or mucus membranes. Sugar scrub should never be applied to the face. Let set for 1 minute, and then gently rise off. Keep in a glass jar with a tight-fitting lid in a cool, dark area for up to 1 month.

Through the Ages Smelling Salts

Smelling salts are something that we think of when we ponder on the Victorian days—back when women wore their corsets so tightly that they would often faint. The salt preserves the oil. Taking a whiff can bring different healing aspects as the oils cross the blood/brain/olfactory barriers. This recipe is great for when you are feeling miserable for days on end, and need a quick pick-me-up at your fingertips.

Yield: ½ teaspoon

RECIPE
1 drop helichrysum oil
1 drop cinnamon oil
1 drop clove oil
½ teaspoon salt

Combine essential oils and salt well with a tiny whisk or fork. Place into a small vial and inhale scent as needed, alternating nostrils. Store in a cool, dark area in a glass vial for up to 1 year.

Passion

Passion is a very strong desire and emotion directed at someone or something. Passion can lead people to do great things: a passion for finding a cure for a disease, the passion to create art, etcetera. Passion can also be a strong emotion in romance. Essential oils, and the plants they derive from, have been used for centuries to increase a person's attraction for another person and bring passion to an all-time high. Increase your passion and do what you were meant to do.

Essential Oils

Cajeput, jasmine, orange, patchouli, rose, sandalwood, and ylang-ylang

I Love You and You Love Me Bath Salts

Help restore your passion for life and people by bathing in these essential oils. This powerful blend contains aphrodisiac, nervine, sedative, and tonic elements and is an old favorite for increasing physical attraction between two people.

Yield: 3 cups

RECIPE

10 drops jasmine oil

5 drops rose oil

5 drops patchouli oil

5 drops vitamin E oil

2 tablespoons carrier oil

3 cups bath salts

1 tablespoon milk (optional for adults, recommended for children)

Use any type of salt you prefer: pink Himalayan salt, sea salt, Epsom salts, etc. In a small container, add the essential oils to the desired type of salt. Stir until well blended. Screw lid onto container tightly. Leave mixture in a dark area for 24 hours and then stir mixture again. Run the bathwater. Once the tub is full of water, you can add the milk, and then add ½ cup of the bath salt mixture to bathwater as you get into the tub. You may stay in the tub as long as the temperature is comfortable. Dry your feet well when you get out of the bath, as the oils are slippery and can cause you to fall. Store remainder in a glass jar or container with a tight-fitting lid in a cool, dark area for up to 3 months. These jars make attractive, inexpensive, and healing gifts!

Alluring Spray

Using these essential oils can bring passion to yourself and those around you. This passion-inducing aroma contains aphrodisiac, nervine, sedative, and antidepressant properties.

Yield: 2 fluid ounces

RECIPE

9 drops rose oil

5 drops patchouli oil

1 tablespoon witch hazel
2 fluid ounces water

Add all ingredients to a dark-colored spray bottle. Check for material steadfastness before spraying on fabric. Shake the bottle and spray onto area desired, such as body, hair, home, car, or office. Do not spray into or on open wounds, genitals, eyes, or mucus membranes. Store in a cool, dark area for up to 3 months. Shake well before each use to combine the ingredients.

Passion Inhale

This essential oil has been used for years in everything from perfume to incense to reportedly attract that soul mate to your life and bring you the passion that you yearn for. Ylang-ylang contains aphrodisiac, euphoric, nervine, tonic, and antidepressant properties.

Yield: 1 application

RECIPE
1 drop ylang-ylang oil

Choose your essential oil and apply to the palm of your hand, an oil inhaler, or a tissue. Bring the essential oils close to your nostrils and inhale the aroma deeply. You can cover one nostril at a time with your thumb and, if you prefer, alternate nostrils. This process sends the properties straight to your brain and the effects are immediate. You can complete this procedure 3–4 times daily.

Passionate Spritzer

Use this blend when you want to inspire, create, and endeavor to bring your artistic side to fruition. Passion to create can be enhanced by using this recipe and spritzing around you when you want to get that passionate creative spark ignited.

Yield: 2 fluid ounces

RECIPE
10 drops orange oil
3 drops jasmine oil

3 drops rose oil

1 tablespoon witch hazel

2 fluid ounces water

Spritzers are lighter than sprays, and easier to wear on the body or in your hair. Mix the essential oils, water, and witch hazel into a spray bottle. Shake well before each use. Lightly spray the area desired, such as body, hair, clothing (check first for color damage to clothing and furniture), rooms, car, or office. The lightly scented fragrance and the healing therapeutic properties will soon make this one of your favorite methods of using your oils. Store the spritzer in a cool, dark area for up to 3 months.

Passion in the Moment

These essential oils will help to ignite a passionate response as well as have a calming and focusing effect on whoever uses it. This recipe contains aphrodisiac, nervine, sedative, and tonic properties.

Yield: 1 fluid ounce

RECIPE

7 drops patchouli oil

5 drops orange oil

3 drops vitamin E oil

1 fluid ounce carrier oil

Pour the essential oils and the carrier oil into a small glass container, bowl, or jar. Swirl to mix the ingredients and use to massage lightly the area desired, such as temples, neck, chest, back, or soles of feet. Keep essential oil mixture away from open wounds, mucus membranes, genitals, eyes, and sensitive areas. Repeat application as needed. Store unused portion in a glass jar or container with a tight-fitting lid in a cool, dark area for up to 3 months.

Lover's Bath

The essential oils combined in this bath recipe can help to create passionate energy. These oils contain aphrodisiac, sedative, antidepressant, and nervine properties.

Yield: 1 application

RECIPE

7 drops rose oil

7 drops jasmine oil

5 drops ylang-ylang oil

1 tablespoon carrier oil

1 tablespoon milk (optional for adults, recommended for children)

As you begin to fill the tub with water, pour the chosen essential oils and carrier oil into the running water. Run a warm, not hot, bath. Water that is too hot will cause the essential oils to dissipate. You may add 1 tablespoon of milk to the water; this ensures that the essential oils will not stick to your skin, but will mix with the water. You may soak in the water as long as you are comfortable. Dry your feet well once you get out of the water, as the oils will cause them to be slippery, increasing your chances of falling. Rinse the tub of any remaining oils.

Paradise Pillow Powder

Sprinkle this essential oil recipe inside your partner's pillow and their thoughts will turn from sleep to loving you and ONLY you with a passion that is undeniable. The therapeutic properties in this blend include aphrodisiac, nervine, sedative, and antidepressant components.

Yield: ½ cup

RECIPE

5 drops rose oil

5 drops jasmine oil

5 drops ylang-ylang oil

4 drops vitamin E oil

½ cup cornstarch

Place the ingredients into a mason jar, stirring well with a whisk. Carefully poke holes into the lid, use this as a shaker, and shake the ingredients into pillowcases or under sheet areas as needed. You can get a piece of plastic wrap and place it over the jar and

under the lid to keep powder from spilling out when not in use. Store in a glass jar or container with a tight-fitting lid in a cool, dark, and dry area for up to 3 months.

Rage

Everybody has feelings of anger, but not everyone experiences fits of rage. Rage is scary and can be very harmful and detrimental to the person acting out and the people who love that person. Mental illness, disease, and heredity play huge factors in rage-filled episodes. These essential oils have been used for years in different ways to help a person learn to keep their rage in check and to learn to express their anger and frustration differently.

Essential Oils

Bergamot, chamomile, clary sage, clove, cypress, frankincense, geranium, jasmine, lavender, mandarin, patchouli, Palo Santo, Roman chamomile, rose, and vetiver

Calming Diffuser

These calming and soothing essential oils can provide the home with an atmosphere of peace. Use this diffuser recipe when tensions are running a little high, and calming influences will surround you.

Yield: 1 application

RECIPE
5 drops clary sage oil
5 drops bergamot oil
Water

Follow your directions for using essential oils in your particular brand of diffuser. Ensure that your diffuser does not use heat but runs by vibration, sound waves, or another cold-steam type of process. Choose the essential oils needed for your condition, then add water and oils to the diffuser. Run your diffuser as needed to permeate the air with therapeutic properties and achieve the results you desire.

Soothing Powder

This powder sprinkled under the sheets is said to soothe and relieve tensions. Try using this blend when emotions are running high and some soothing bliss is needed. Calming and soothing properties help to achieve peace and sleep.

Yield: ¼ cup

RECIPE
8 drops vetiver oil
3 drops chamomile oil
3 drops lavender oil
¼ cup cornstarch
4 drops vitamin E oil

Place the ingredients into a mason jar, stirring well with a whisk. Carefully poke holes into the lid, use this as a shaker, and shake the ingredients into pillowcases or under sheet areas as needed. You can get a piece of plastic wrap and place it over the jar and under the lid to keep powder from spilling out when not in use. Store in a glass jar or container with a tight-fitting lid in a cool, dark, and dry area for up to 3 months.

Smile Spray

This spray uses essential oils that have a calming, uplifting effect. Try spraying this on your linens, clothing, car, or office. You can handle anything with a smile after soaking up these scents.

Yield: 2 fluid ounces

RECIPE
9 drops cypress oil
9 drops rose oil
5 drops jasmineoil
1 fluid ounce distilled water
1 fluid ounce vodka

Add all ingredients to a dark-colored spray bottle. Check for material steadfastness before spraying on fabric. Shake the bottle and spray onto area desired, such as body,

hair, home, car, or office. Do not spray into or on open wounds, genitals, eyes, or mucus membranes. Store in a cool, dark area for up to 1 year. Shake well before each use to combine the ingredients.

Calm, Cool, and Collected Salve

This recipe has essential oils known for their calming therapeutic properties. Wear this salve before going into a situation in which you need to remain calm and cool.

Yield: 1 tablespoon

RECIPE
7 drops clary sage oil
5 drops jasmine oil
3 drops mandarin oil
1 teaspoon beeswax pellets
4 drops vitamin E oil
3 teaspoons carrier oil

Heat the beeswax and the carrier oil in a glass bowl in the microwave for 1 ½–2 minutes, until just melted, or on low on the stovetop. If you open the door every 15 seconds, you can avoid the popping of the wax and oil and overheating. Carefully remove the container from the microwave and stir. Drip a drop of the melted oil and wax onto the counter, after 1 minute check for consistency. If it is too thin, add more beeswax to the container; if it is too thick, add more carrier oil. Add the vitamin E oil and the essential oil to the heated mixture in the container. Whisk lightly, and it will begin hardening immediately. Pour into containers. Ensure your containers are glass or tin to prevent leeching of chemicals. Once cool, apply to wrists, temples, neck, or soles of feet. Do not apply to mucus membranes, eyes, genitals, or open wounds. Label containers and store in a dark, dry area for up to 1 year.

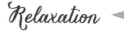

Relaxation

Relaxation is one of the things that most of us live for. That vacation we look forward to all year, a few hours sitting on the porch at sunset, relaxing with a cup of coffee in the morning—it makes everything all worth it. Relaxation is a multibillion-dollar industry in America. You can have a very special private place of zen and relaxation in your own home or office by incorporating your own essential oils into your relaxation process. There are so many calming, sedating, tranquilizing essential oils that it is hard to just choose a few to try.

Essential Oils

Bergamot, cedarwood, clary sage, fennel, frankincense, German chamomile, jasmine, lavender, lemon, marjoram, neroli, patchouli, Roman chamomile, rose, sandalwood, vetiver, and ylang-ylang

Floating Cloud Powder

Look at the list of essential oils in this recipe; each one brings a sense of calm just by looking at the name. Luxuriating in a bed that has been sprinkled with this powder is like resting on a cloud. The relaxing properties of these oils contain antidepressant, nervine, sedative, and calming agents.

Yield: ¼ cup

RECIPE
5 drops German chamomile oil
5 drops Roman chamomile oil
3 drops lavender oil
2 drops vetiver oil
4 drops vitamin E oil
¼ cup cornstarch

Place the ingredients into a mason jar, stirring well with a whisk. Carefully poke holes into the lid, use this as a shaker, and shake the ingredients into pillowcases or under sheet areas as needed. You can get a piece of plastic wrap and place it over the jar and under the lid to keep powder from spilling out when not in use. Store in a glass jar or container with a tight-fitting lid in a cool, dark, and dry area for up to 3 months.

Spring Rejuvenating Bath Salts

Not only do the chamomile oils relax you, but the bergamot oil heals and protects you as you soak up all the relaxation you desire. The jasmine oil is full of calming properties and also imparts an aroma that you won't soon forget. The healing and calming properties of this recipe include analgesic, antidepressant, anti-inflammatory, sedative, and nervine components.

Yield: 3 cups

RECIPE

7 drops German chamomile oil

5 drops Roman chamomile oil

5 drops bergamot oil

3 drops jasmine oil

4 drops vitamin E oil

2 tablespoons carrier oil

3 cups salt

1 tablespoon milk (optional for adults, recommended for children)

Use any type of salt you prefer: pink Himalayan salt, sea salt, Epsom salts, etc. In a small container, add the essential oils to the desired type of salt. Stir until well blended. Screw lid onto container tightly. Leave mixture in a dark area for 24 hours and then stir mixture again. Run the bathwater. Once the tub is full of water, you can add the milk, and then add ½ cup of the bath salt mixture to bathwater as you get into the tub. You may stay in the tub as long as the temperature is comfortable. Dry your feet well when you get out of the bath, as the oils are slippery and can cause you to fall. Store remainder in a glass jar or container with a tight-fitting lid in a cool, dark area for up to 3 months. These jars make attractive, inexpensive, and healing gifts!

Om Diffuser

This is a perfect blend of essential oils for relaxation and meditation. I just can't get enough of these aromas or the sense of calm that surrounds me as I luxuriate in the air of this blend. The calming properties of this recipe include antidepressant, anti-irritability and nervous tension, sedative, and restorative elements.

Yield: 1 application

RECIPE
5 drops lavender oil
5 drops bergamot oil
2 drops neroli oil
Water

Follow your directions for using essential oils in your particular brand of diffuser. Ensure that your diffuser does not use heat but runs by vibration, sound waves, or another cold-steam type of process. Choose the essential oils needed for your condition, then add water and oils to the diffuser. Run your diffuser as needed to permeate the air with therapeutic properties and achieve the results you desire.

Instant Calm in a Bottle

These essential oils will provide you with instant relaxation when you are dealing with stressful outside influences. Bring in all of the positive influences in your life by inhaling these scents. The properties of these oils contain calming, sedative, and anti-depressant components.

Yield: 1 application

RECIPE
1 drop lavender oil
or
1 drop cedarwood oil
or
1 drop chamomile oil

Choose your essential oil and apply to the palm of your hand, an oil inhaler, or a tissue. Bring the essential oils close to your nostrils and inhale the aroma deeply. You can cover one nostril at a time with your thumb and, if you prefer, alternate nostrils. This process sends the properties straight to your brain and the effects are immediate. You can complete this procedure 3–4 times daily.

Cruise to Nowhere Bath

The essential oils in this bath recipe will have you relaxing so much you will think you are on a luxury yacht sailing to the Bahamas. Take the trip of a lifetime right in the comfort of your own home with this "sail me away" comforting recipe. This blend incorporates antidepressant, aphrodisiac, depurative, nervine, and sedative properties.

Yield: 1 application

RECIPE

5 drops bergamot oil

5 drops cedarwood oil

5 drops rose oil

5 drops lavender oil

1 tablespoon milk (optional for adults, recommended for children)

As you begin to fill the tub with water, pour the chosen essential oils and carrier oil into the running water. Run a warm, not hot, bath. Water that is too hot will cause the essential oils to dissipate. You may add 1 tablespoon of milk to the water; this ensures that the essential oils will not stick to your skin, but will mix with the water. You may soak in the water as long as you are comfortable. Dry your feet well once you get out of the water, as the oils will cause them to be slippery, increasing your chances of falling. Rinse the tub of any remaining oils.

Ancient Wonders Spray

If you are feeling agitated or anxious, this spray will calm your mood and give you that chilled-out attitude. These oils have been used since ancient times to bring calm and peace to the inhaler. These essential oils contain sedative, antidepressant, relaxing, and calming properties.

Yield: 2 fluid ounces

RECIPE

11 drops lavender oil

5 drops rose oil

4 drops bergamot oil

1 tablespoon witch hazel

2 fluid ounces water

Add all ingredients to a dark-colored spray bottle. Check for material steadfastness before spraying on fabric. Shake the bottle and spray onto area desired, such as body, hair, home, car, or office. Do not spray into or on open wounds, genitals, eyes, or mucus membranes. Store in a cool, dark area for up to 3 months. Shake well before each use to combine the ingredients.

Mind-Blowing Massage

Get the best massage of your life by incorporating these oils into your massage. The elements at work in this blend include sedative, aphrodisiac, antidepressant, and nervine properties to give you the relaxation you are searching for.

Yield: 1 fluid ounce

RECIPE

4 drops lavender oil

5 drops bergamot oil

4 drops rose oil

3 drops vitamin E oil

1 fluid ounce carrier oil

Pour the essential oils and the carrier oil into a small glass container, bowl, or jar. Swirl to mix the ingredients and use to massage lightly the area desired, such as temples, neck, chest, back, or soles of feet. Keep essential oil mixture away from open wounds, mucus membranes, genitals, eyes, and sensitive areas. Repeat application as needed. Store unused portion in a glass jar or container with a tight-fitting lid in a cool, dark area for up to 3 months.

Remorse

Everyone has, at some time in their life, done something that filled them with deep guilt and a longing to change what happened. We say words thoughtlessly, commit actions that are otherwise unconscionable, and hurt those we love. Staying in the frame of mind that remorse puts us in can greatly affect other aspects of our lives, such as our health and our relationships. If apologizing or another action cannot change the thing you have done, then it is time to forgive yourself, heal, and vow to make up for that action in a better, more positive way. Healing your remorse with essential oils, prayer, and self-forgiveness are practices that you can do alone, and you can do them effectively.

Essential Oils

Angelica, cedarwood, cypress, frankincense, lavender, linden blossom, melissa, sage, and sandalwood

Forgiveness Powder

Sleeping on this powder of healing essential oils will help you on the path of forgiving and trusting yourself again. These oils reportedly calm your mind, reduce anxiety, and help you to have a guilt-free night's sleep.

Yield: ¼ cup

RECIPE
5 drops cedarwood oil
5 drops sage oil
5 drops angelica oil
4 drops vitamin E oil
¼ cup cornstarch

Place the ingredients into a mason jar, stirring well with a whisk. Carefully poke holes into the lid, use this as a shaker, and shake the ingredients into pillowcases or under sheet areas as needed. You can get a piece of plastic wrap and place it over the jar and

under the lid to keep powder from spilling out when not in use. Store in a glass jar or container with a tight-fitting lid in a cool, dark, and dry area for up to 3 months.

Sincere Apology Diffuser

These are the essential oils I once used to help me get through a very hard apology with a friend. These oils gave me the strength to apologize with conviction and inner healing for my soul. These aromas helped my friend to open her heart and accept my apology with love and forgiveness, even if I felt I didn't deserve it.

Yield: 1 application

RECIPE
3 drops frankincense oil
3 drops sandalwood oil
3 drops melissa oil
2 drops linden blossom oil
Water

Follow your directions for using essential oils in your particular brand of diffuser. Ensure that your diffuser does not use heat but runs by vibration, sound waves, or another cold-steam type of process. Choose the essential oils needed for your condition, then add water and oils to the diffuser. Run your diffuser as needed to permeate the air with therapeutic properties and achieve the results you desire.

Forgiveness Footbath

This footbath releases oils into the air and into the body that can have you not only forgiving yourself, but your heart will be open enough to forgive others as well. The warm, relaxing water and the antianxiety properties of these oils will have you feeling contentment and peace once again.

Yield: 1 application

RECIPE
5 drops neroli oil
4 drops lavender oil

4 drops cypress oil

3 drops sage oil

1 tablespoon milk (optional for adults, recommended for children)

Warm water

Combine the oils, milk, and any other ingredients into a container large enough to comfortably rest your feet. Fill the container at least halfway with water that is not too hot, but as hot as you can comfortably stand it. Gently submerge your feet in the water and sit back and relax. Leave your feet in the footbath until the water is cool or uncomfortable, about 15 minutes. Dry feet and feel the energized peace you receive from this luxurious spa treatment. Discard water.

Sadness

When someone you love is surrounded by an aura of sadness, it affects not only them, but everyone who loves them. Sadness can permeate our thoughts, work, health, relationships, and every other part of our lives. Using essential oils to open one's heart and spirit to joy is a long-held practice of many cultures. By inundating a person's home or other space with healing essential oils, we can give our loved ones a chance of opening up to happiness again. These oils affect chemicals in our brains that promote endorphins, excitement, and joy.

Essential Oils

Cardamom, cedarwood, clary sage, clove, frankincense, geranium, ginseng, grapefruit, jasmine, juniper berry, lavender, neroli, orange, Palma Rosa, Palo Santo, peppermint, rose, and spearmint

Work It Out Diffuser

Who can help but feel a small uplifting of the spirit with these aromas wafting throughout the home? I love these bright, happy oils and use them often to dispel the gloom of a family member when they are feeling sad.

Yield: 1 application

RECIPE
2 drops spearmint oil
2 drops bergamot oil
2 drops grapefruit oil
Water

Follow your directions for using essential oils in your particular brand of diffuser. Ensure that your diffuser does not use heat but runs by vibration, sound waves, or another cold-steam type of process. Choose the essential oils needed for your condition, then add water and oils to the diffuser. Run your diffuser as needed to permeate the air with therapeutic properties and achieve the results you desire.

Bath and Shower Gift Bombs

Use these shower and bath bombs as presents for those you love, and they will receive happiness, not only from the gift, but from the powerful uplifting properties of the oils that the bombs are laden with. They will love the fizzle and smells of the bath bombs, and the natural feel-good properties of these oils cling to them and brighten up their day.

Yield: 8–12 bombs

RECIPE
1 cup baking soda
½ cup citric acid
½ cup cornstarch
½ cup Epsom salts, fine grained
15 drops juniper berry oil
15 drops Palo Santo oil
5 drops lavender oil
½ teaspoon carrier oil
¾ teaspoon water
spray bottle (water)

In a large bowl, mix your dry ingredients together until fine with a whisk. In a tiny jar with a lid, add your wet ingredients and shake to mix. You may add a couple drops of food coloring to the wet jar. Extremely slowly, add the wet ingredients to the dry ingredients while whisking rapidly. If fizzing takes place, whisk until it is mixed. Once the ingredients are well mixed, it should be the texture of slightly damp sand. Add a spray or two of water if needed. Once the mixture is the consistency you like, form into balls; I just smash mine down into ice cube trays or muffin tins. You can use cute molds, but you must work rapidly as mixture will dry out quickly. Leave in open air, uncovered, in a room where they will not be disturbed for 12–24 hours. Once they are dry, you can place 1–2 bombs into your bath or directly into the spray of the shower and they will fizz and release their aromatic and healing properties. Store unused portion in an airtight container for up to 6 months.

Silky Sheet Spray

If you have ever suffered from all-consuming sadness, you know the place you want to be more than anywhere else is in bed. When you are sad, it's your thought process that needs changing. Becoming a part of the solution to a problem can start by using this recipe on yourself. Use this uplifting spray to help turn those negative thoughts into happy thoughts and make the bed a place where you can recharge your soul and dispel any sadness.

Yield: 2 fluid ounces

RECIPE
5 drops bergamot oil
5 drops eucalyptus oil
5 drops juniper berry oil
1 fluid ounce distilled water
1 fluid ounce vodka

Add all ingredients to a dark-colored spray bottle. Check for material steadfastness before spraying on fabric. Shake the bottle and spray onto area desired, such as body, hair, home, car, or office. Do not spray into or on open wounds, genitals, eyes, or mucus membranes. Store in a cool, dark area for up to 3 months. Shake well before each use to combine the ingredients.

Shame

Feelings of shame can be slight or significant, depending on each individual situation. Shame can come from not only feeling distress or mortification about something you have done or caused, but also by being in a situation that causes you to feel embarrassment or indignity. Overcoming feelings of shame is something that we have to work on within ourselves. We can ask for forgiveness, not repeat an action, or not let situations out of our control affect us so deeply. These essential oils are meant to bring joy into your life and fill you with positivity and hope to get you over the shame you are feeling.

Essential Oils

Allspice, bitter orange, calendula, cardamom, fennel, geranium, ginger, holy basil, jasmine, lemongrass, lime, lotus, nutmeg, palmarosa, Palo Santo, petitgrain, spearmint, and ylang-ylang

I'm So Sorry Lotion

I wear this lotion when I am in the process of apologizing or healing myself. I want to be fair in my apologies and have a clear assessment of the situation. These oils help me to communicate my thoughts, put me at ease, and also put the person I am with at ease as well, so that we can be open and truthful with each other about the situation at hand.

Yield: 1 fluid ounce

RECIPE
3 drops petitgrain oil
3 drops spearmint oil
2 drops rosewood oil
1 fluid ounce unscented body lotion

Add the recommended amount of essential oils to any brand of mild unscented lotion. Whisk until thoroughly mixed. Apply lotion to body as needed. Store unused portion in a jar with a tight-fitting lid in a cool, dark area for up to 3 months.

I Forgive Me Spray

It is harder for us to forgive ourselves than it is for others to forgive us. Sometimes shame can be with a person many years, or even decades, after the event that caused the shame. Forgiving oneself can ease the shame and guilt we feel. These essential oils help us to love ourselves and get over the self-inflicted indignity we heap upon ourselves in our own minds.

Yield: 2 fluid ounces

RECIPE

8 drops petitgrain oil

5 drops palmarosa oil

3 drops jasmine oil

3 drops ylang-ylang oil

1 tablespoon witch hazel

2 fluid ounces water

Add all ingredients to a dark-colored spray bottle. Check for material steadfastness before spraying on fabric. Shake the bottle and spray onto area desired, such as body, hair, home, car, or office. Do not spray into or on open wounds, genitals, eyes, or mucus membranes. Store in a cool, dark area for up to 3 months. Shake well before each use to combine the ingredients.

CHAPTER 5
Recipes for Needs

This chapter deals with needs that everyone has in their lives from time to time. We all have areas of ourselves that we would like to improve or eliminate. These recipes can give you that added boost you need when trying to better yourself on your journey through life.

Balance

Many people try to find a balance in their own personal chaos due to having too many areas of their lives out of sync. These can include career, family, illness, spirituality, money issues, and numerous other concerns. Any little thing can be the tipping factor in how our day goes. We can be thrown into anxiety, fear, anger, stress, and devastation so easily when we are out of balance. These essential oils have shown throughout the ages that they have the ability to help us to achieve that balance that we all so desperately need by increasing focus, calm, and truth within ourselves.

Essential Oils

Cedarwood, clary sage, cypress, eucalyptus, geranium, jasmine, lavender, melissa, Roman chamomile, vetiver, and ylang-ylang

Life-Balancing Powder

These essential oils are from herbs long associated with balancing one's life. When the chaos gets to be too much, sleep on this therapeutic powder made from essential oils that will have you waking up to the feeling that you can accomplish anything. The balancing properties of this blend include antidepressant, nervine, and euphoric functions that will have you feeling great and assist you in making wise decisions.

Yield: ¼ cup

RECIPE
3 drops jasmine oil
3 drops clary sage oil
3 drops geranium oil
¼ cup cornstarch
4 drops vitamin E oil

Place the ingredients into a mason jar, stirring well with a whisk. Carefully poke holes into the lid, use this as a shaker, and shake the ingredients into pillowcases or under sheet areas as needed. You can get a piece of plastic wrap and place it over the jar and under the lid to keep powder from spilling out when not in use. Store in a glass jar or container with a tight-fitting lid in a cool, dark, and dry area for up to 3 months.

Balancing Inhaler

When your thoughts are in chaos, bring them back into balance by smelling this essential oil blend's aroma. The oils in this recipe contain sedative, calming, and euphoric properties that will have you feeling like YOU again.

Yield: 1 application

RECIPE
2 drops cedarwood oil
2 drops ylang-ylang oil

Choose your essential oil and apply to the palm of your hand, an oil inhaler, or a tissue. Bring the essential oils close to your nostrils and inhale the aroma deeply. You can

cover one nostril at a time with your thumb and, if you prefer, alternate nostrils. This process sends the properties straight to your brain and the effects are immediate. You can complete this process 3–4 times daily.

Balancing Bath

Bath salts always seem to bring me back into balance, but when you add these essential oils, you will feel you can handle anything with a smile. The mood-lifting properties of these essential oils are euphoric, tonic, stimulating, and calming for life balance.

Yield: 3 cups

RECIPE

6 drops vetiver oil

6 drops jasmine oil

6 drops clary sage oil

2 drops lavender oil

3 cups salt

1 tablespoon carrier oil

1 tablespoon milk (optional for adults, recommended for children)

Use any type of salt you prefer: pink Himalayan salt, sea salt, Epsom salts, etc. In a small container, add the essential oils to the desired type of salt. Stir until well blended. Screw lid onto container tightly. Leave mixture in a dark area for 24 hours and then stir mixture again. Run the bathwater. Once the tub is full of water, you can add the milk, and then add ½ cup of the bath salt mixture to bathwater as you get into the tub. You may stay in the tub as long as the temperature is comfortable. Dry your feet well when you get out of the bath, as the oils are slippery and can cause you to fall. Store remainder in a glass jar or container with a tight-fitting lid in a cool, dark area for up to 3 months. These jars make attractive, inexpensive, and healing gifts!

Concentration

The inability to focus for extended periods of time is a lack of concentration. There are many mitigating circumstances that could cause a person to be unable to retain the ability to concentrate. Essential oils often can increase the focus and concentration of a person, as well as increase their memory. Whether you have a huge task before you, a project you need to focus on, or something else that needs your complete attention, these recipes will help you to get a leg up on your concentration.

Essential Oils

Basil, bergamot, cedarwood, peppermint, rose, rosemary, spearmint, and vetiver

Winning Massage Oil

The essential oils in this recipe have long been used to sharpen focus and concentration. The therapeutic properties in this blend contain tonic, purifying, nervine, and mental fatigue clearing elements. I need this massage oil often—especially the massage part! These oils work when I know I am going to be at my computer all day and I need to get a lot of laser-focused work done.

Yield: 2–6 applications

RECIPE
5 drops cedarwood oil
3 drops bergamot oil
2 drops rose oil
2 drops basil oil
4 drops vitamin E oil
2 tablespoons carrier oil

Pour the essential oils and the carrier oil into a small glass container, bowl, or jar. Swirl to mix the ingredients and use to massage lightly the area desired, such as temples, neck, chest, back, or soles of feet. Keep essential oil mixture away from open wounds, mucus membranes, genitals, eyes, and sensitive areas. Repeat application as needed. Store unused portion in a glass jar or container with a tight-fitting lid in a cool, dark area for up to 3 months.

Focus in the Air Diffuser

This diffuser will help you to keep everyone in the household or the office focused on tasks that need to be completed. These essential oils have long been known to promote memory and focus with their cephalic, invigorating, and stimulating properties. This will also give everyone a little energy boost, which is much needed in our hectic society.

Yield: 1 application

RECIPE
2 drops peppermint oil
2 drops rose oil
2 drops bergamot oil
Water

Follow your directions for using essential oils in your particular brand of diffuser. Ensure that your diffuser does not use heat but runs by vibration, sound waves, or another cold-steam type of process. Choose the essential oils needed for your condition, then add water and oils to the diffuser. Run your diffuser as needed to permeate the air with therapeutic properties and achieve the results you desire.

Single-Mindedness Bath Salts

When you need to focus all of your attention on one subject, relax in this bath with these powerful essential oils reported to help you keep your thoughts on where they need to be. You will come out of the bath ready to tackle that task. The stimulating, tonic, and restorative properties in these essential oils will get your mind sharp and focused and infuse your body with energy.

Yield: 3 cups

RECIPE
5 drops rosemary oil
5 drops vetiver oil

    5 drops rose oil

    5 drops bergamot oil

    2 tablespoons carrier oil

    4 drops vitamin E oil

    3 cups bath salts

    1 tablespoon milk (optional for adults, recommended for children)

Use any type of salt you prefer: pink Himalayan salt, sea salt, Epsom salts, etc. In a small container, add the essential oils to the desired type of salt. Stir until well blended. Screw lid onto container tightly. Leave mixture in a dark area for 24 hours and then stir mixture again. Run the bathwater. Once the tub is full of water, you can add the milk, and then add ½ cup of the bath salt mixture to bathwater as you get into the tub. You may stay in the tub as long as the temperature is comfortable. Dry your feet well when you get out of the bath, as the oils are slippery and can cause you to fall. Store remainder in a glass jar or container with a tight-fitting lid in a cool, dark area for up to 3 months. These jars make attractive, inexpensive, and healing gifts!

Focus Lip Balm

When you need to have your wits about you and you want an extra added boost of focus, this is the blend for you. This lip balm has therapeutic properties that have been used for focus and concentration with great results.

    Yield: 1 tablespoon

    RECIPE

    3 teaspoons grape seed oil

    ½ teaspoon beeswax pellets

    4 drops vitamin E oil

    3 drops peppermint oil

    3 drops pink bergamot oil

Melt the beeswax and the carrier oil in a glass bowl in the microwave until most of the beeswax is melted. You can also use a pan on the stovetop on low. Cool slightly. Add the vitamin E and the essential oils and stir or whisk quickly. With a spoon, drip a drop of the mixture onto the counter and Let set for 1 minute. Pull your finger through the drop and check for consistency. If mixture is too thin, add more beeswax; if it is too thick, add more oil. Once desired consistency is acquired, immediately pour into small balm container (glass or metal) with a lid. After mixture cools, cover and store in a cool, dark area for up to 6 months.

Eyes on the Prize Lotion

When you need to concentrate on a single goal or outcome, make sure you first use this lotion blend that has the essential oils reported to help focus and concentration.

Yield: 1 fluid ounce

RECIPE

3 drops rose oil

3 drops bergamot oil

2 drops rosemary oil

1 fluid ounce unscented body lotion

Add the recommended amount of essential oils to any brand of mild unscented lotion. Whisk until thoroughly mixed. Apply lotion to body as needed. Store unused portion in a jar with a tight-fitting lid in a cool, dark area for up to 3 months.

Empathy

Having worked in the social work field for most of my life, I have quite a developed sense of empathy. This is the ability to feel how another person feels, or to understand their emotions, whether you personally agree with their choices or not. Sometimes people have little empathy toward others; we can work on increasing this emotion through essential oils. I like to permeate a room with these aromas and empathy-producing oils when I am working for a charity fund or needing others for volunteer help!

Essential Oils

Cajuput, lavender, lemon, peppermint, pine, wild orange, and ylang-ylang

Empathy Diffuser

These oils will help you to open your mind and feel others on a deeper and a more personal level. Your friends and family will be more sensitive to your plight, and you to theirs, if these oils are wafting through the air. The aromatic properties in this blend work well together to give us a deeper understanding of others, calm us, and help us to listen with an open heart and mind.

Yield: 1 application

RECIPE
5 drops wild orange oil
4 drops pine oil
Water

Follow your directions for using essential oils in your particular brand of diffuser. Ensure that your diffuser does not use heat but runs by vibration, sound waves, or another cold-steam type of process. Choose the essential oils needed for your condition, then add water and oils to the diffuser. Run your diffuser as needed to permeate the air with therapeutic properties and achieve the results you desire.

Open-Minded Spray

I like to spray this when I am trying to talk to others about helping me with a project that will benefit many. I am prone to volunteer and perform charity functions when asked, and with this spray, I find people are more open and receptive to assisting. The therapeutic properties include calming, sedative, aphrodisiac, euphoric, nervine, and tonic components.

Yield: 2 fluid ounces

RECIPE
9 drops lavender oil
7 drops ylang-ylang oil
4 drops cajuput oil
1 tablespoon witch hazel
2 fluid ounces water

Add all ingredients to a dark-colored spray bottle. Check for material steadfastness before spraying on fabric. Shake the bottle and spray onto area desired. Do not spray into or on open wounds, genitals, eyes, or mucus membranes. Store in a cool, dark area for up to 3 months. Shake well before each use to combine the ingredients.

Empathetic Bath and Shower Bombs

These oils are full of calming and soothing natural elements that will give you the ability to relax, listen, and empathize with someone you really have never seen eye-to-eye with. Take this bath when you want to be more open and empathetic.

Yield: 12–18 balls

RECIPE

1 cup baking soda

½ cup citric acid

½ cup cornstarch

½ cup Epsom salts, fine grained

15 drops lemon oil

15 drops peppermint oil

½ teaspoon carrier oil

¾ teaspoon water

spray bottle (water)

In a large bowl, mix your dry ingredients together until fine with a whisk. In a tiny jar with a lid, add your wet ingredients and shake to mix. You may add a couple drops of food coloring to the wet jar. Extremely slowly, add the wet ingredients to the dry ingredients while whisking rapidly. If fizzing takes place, whisk until it is mixed. Once the ingredients are well mixed, it should be the texture of slightly damp sand. Add a spray or two of water if needed. Once the mixture is the consistency you like, form into balls; I just smash mine down into ice cube trays or muffin tins. You can use cute molds, but you must work rapidly as mixture will dry out quickly. Leave in open air, uncovered, in a room where they will not be disturbed for 12–24 hours. Once they are dry, you can place 1–2 bombs into your bath or directly into the spray of the shower and they will fizz and release their aromatic and healing properties. Store unused portion in an airtight container for up to 6 months.

Encouragement

When you need that added boost of confidence from someone else and they are just not giving it, it can dash your self-esteem and have you feeling like maybe you can't complete your task. These essential oils can build you up with encouragement, and can also prompt others to be more encouraging toward you. When you have too much to do to encourage your family members in their efforts in something, these oils will open you up to being more empathetic toward them when they need it most.

Essential Oils

Black pepper, basil, cedarwood, geranium, grapefruit, lavender, sandalwood, and vetiver

You Can Do It Spray

This spray can be used anywhere, anytime. It's so handy when you need that little nudge to get you to take that first step. Feel yourself becoming more confident and self-assured after spraying yourself with this blend containing calming, focusing, and aromatic properties.

Yield: 2 fluid ounces

RECIPE

9 drops vetiver oil

9 drops geranium oil

1 tablespoon witch hazel

4 drops vitamin E oil

2 fluid ounces water

Add all ingredients to a dark-colored spray bottle. Check for material steadfastness before spraying on fabric. Shake the bottle and spray onto area desired. Do not spray into or on open wounds, genitals, eyes, or mucus membranes. Store in a cool, dark area for up to 3 months. Shake well before each use to combine the ingredients.

Tell Me Something Good

Permeate your home with encouraging aromas that will help you to have confidence in yourself and give yourself that positive thinking that you need right now.

Yield: 1 application

RECIPE
5 drops cedarwood oil
5 drops grapefruit oil
4 drops basil oil
Water

Follow your directions for using essential oils in your particular brand of diffuser. Ensure that your diffuser does not use heat but runs by vibration, sound waves, or another cold-steam type of process. Choose the essential oils needed for your condition, then add water and oils to the diffuser. Run your diffuser as needed to permeate the air with therapeutic properties and achieve the results you desire.

Encouragement Lotion

When you want to ensure that your listening skills are at their best and that you can be fully present for someone else, use this beautiful aroma on your skin. Get better focused and able to help someone when under the influence of these calming and focusing oils.

Yield: 1 fluid ounce

RECIPE
3 drops lavender oil
3 drops grapefruit oil
2 drops vetiver oil
1 fluid ounce unscented body lotion

Add the recommended amount of essential oils to any brand of mild unscented lotion. Whisk until thoroughly mixed. Apply lotion to body as needed. Store unused portion in a jar with a tight-fitting lid in a cool, dark area for up to 3 months.

Endurance

Endurance is the ability to forge onward despite obstacles. Essential oils can help a person with the desire and the ability to persist and endure. We often let life get in the way of our dreams and goals. We can endure those obstacles and achieve what we want, even if we need outside help such as essential oils. Prayer, meditation, and spiritual work are often used by those capable of enduring the pitfalls of life. Essential oils can work wonders in helping you to persist despite the odds.

Essential Oils

Black pepper, lemongrass, rosemary, and sandalwood

Loving Linen Powder

These essential oils are reported to increase endurance with their energy-enhancing and aphrodisiacal qualities. Sprinkle them under the sheets and into the pillowcases for a long night of vitality and endurance.

Yield: ¼ cup

RECIPE
3 drops rosemary oil
3 drops sandalwood oil
3 drops lemongrass oil
4 drops vitamin E oil
¼ cup cornstarch

Place the ingredients into a mason jar, stirring well with a whisk. Carefully poke holes into the lid, use this as a shaker, and shake the ingredients into pillowcases or under sheet areas as needed. You can get a piece of plastic wrap and place it over the jar and under the lid to keep powder from spilling out when not in use. Store in a glass jar or container with a tight-fitting lid in a cool, dark, and dry area for up to 3 months.

Ever-Enduring Bath

When facing the day, we often feel we will be unable to endure what we know is ahead of us … tasks, phone calls, paperwork—it just goes on and on and on. These oils are reported to build up stamina, energy, and endurance. Soak in this bath and you will have the energy and wherewithal to go all day or all night long.

Yield: 1 application

RECIPE
2 drops black pepper oil
6 drops lemongrass oil
6 drops sandalwood oil
1 tablespoon carrier oil
1 tablespoon milk (optional for adults, recommended for children)

As you begin to fill the tub with water, pour the chosen essential oils and carrier oil into the running water. Run a warm, not hot, bath. Water that is too hot will cause the essential oils to dissipate. You may add 1 tablespoon of milk to the water; this ensures that the essential oils will not stick to your skin, but will mix with the water. You may soak in the water as long as you are comfortable. Dry your feet well once you get out of the water, as the oils will cause them to be slippery, increasing your chances of falling. Rinse the tub of any remaining oils.

Filled with Energy Massage

When you know you have an upcoming event that is going to sap all of your strength and energy, prepare ahead of time by using these essential oils reputed to provide endurance and power to get you through that task. These energy-inducing therapeutic properties can help you to withstand anything they throw at you.

Yield: 1–2 applications

RECIPE
5 drops sandalwood oil
1 drop black pepper oil
3 drops vitamin E oil
1 tablespoon carrier oil

Pour the essential oils and the carrier oil into a small glass container, bowl, or jar. Swirl to mix the ingredients and use to massage lightly the area desired, such as temples, neck, chest, back, or soles of feet. Keep essential oil mixture away from open wounds, mucus membranes, genitals, eyes, and sensitive areas. Repeat application as needed. Store unused portion in a glass jar or container with a tight-fitting lid in a cool, dark area for up to 3 months.

Diffuser of Persistence

This is the diffuser I run if I have a whole day of chores to do inside of my home. I just put a couple of drops of these oils into the diffuser, turn on the music, and go till I can't go anymore. The energizing properties help me to achieve all of my goals and have fun while doing it.

Yield: 1 application

RECIPE
3 drops lemongrass oil
3 drops sandalwood oil
Water

Follow your directions for using essential oils in your particular brand of diffuser. Ensure that your diffuser does not use heat but runs by vibration, sound waves, or another cold-steam type of process. Choose the essential oils needed for your condition, then add water and oils to the diffuser. Run your diffuser as needed to permeate the air with therapeutic properties and achieve the results you desire.

Enduring Inhaler

Carry a couple vials of these essential oils with you for an instant burst of longevity and endurance. The aromas are great and are full of energy-boosting properties.

Yield: 1 application

RECIPE
1 drop lemongrass oil
or
1 drop sandalwood oil

Choose your essential oil and apply to the palm of your hand, an oil inhaler, or a tissue. Bring the essential oils close to your nostrils and inhale the aroma deeply. You can cover one nostril at a time with your thumb and, if you prefer, alternate nostrils. This process sends the properties straight to your brain and the effects are immediate. You can complete this process 3–4 times daily.

Endurance Bath Salts

The essential oils in this recipe are perfect for getting you ready to go another day, all day long. This recipe is chock-full of long-lasting, endurance-promoting essential oils.

Yield: 3 cups

RECIPE

5 drops rosemary oil

5 drops sandalwood oil

6 drops lemongrass oil

2 tablespoons carrier oil

5 drops vitamin E oil

3 cups salts

1 tablespoon milk (optional for adults, recommended for children)

Use any type of salt you prefer: pink Himalayan salt, sea salt, Epsom salts, etc. In a small container, add the essential oils to the desired type of salt. Stir until well blended. Screw lid onto container tightly. Leave mixture in a dark area for 24 hours and then stir mixture again. Run the bathwater. Once the tub is full of water, you can add the milk, and then add ½ cup of the bath salt mixture to bathwater as you get into the tub. These jars make attractive, inexpensive, and healing gifts! Store remainder in a glass jar or container with a tight-fitting lid in a cool, dark area for up to 3 months.

Forge Ahead Spray

Use this spray to give yourself that boost you need when you find your energy is flagging. These essential oils are reportedly great for increasing stamina and boosting power.

Yield: 2 fluid ounces

RECIPE
9 drops sandalwood oil
4 drops lemongrass oil
3 drops rosemary oil
2 drops black pepper oil
1 tablespoon witch hazel
2 fluid ounces water

Add all ingredients to a dark-colored spray bottle. Check for material steadfastness before spraying on fabric. Shake the bottle and spray onto area desired, such as body, hair, home, car, or office. Do not spray into or on open wounds, genitals, eyes, or mucus membranes. Store in a cool, dark area for up to 3 months. Shake well before each use to combine the ingredients.

Energy

Energy is something that usually comes from within a person. Sometimes people suffering from depression, fatigue, heartbreak, grief, and illness find that they have a lack of energy and do not have the desire to even complete the most mundane of tasks. Essential oils can help a person regain the energy to join the outside world and forge ahead. Or if, like me, you just want an additional energy boost to clean the house or complete a project, these blends will work just as well for you.

Essential Oils

Basil, bergamot, black pepper, eucalyptus, cinnamon, clove, cypress, frankincense, fir, grapefruit, lemon, lemongrass, patchouli, peppermint, patchouli, and sage

Energy Power Boosting Inhale

The quick boost you need to get you through that "one more thing" that you must accomplish is readily available for you. The energizing ability of this recipe is due to the tonic and stimulating properties in these essential oils. I love to take a whiff of these oils when I have a quick need of instant energy and enthusiasm to complete something.

Yield: 1 application

RECIPE
1 drop lemon oil

or

1 drop peppermint oil

or

1 drop pine oil

Choose your essential oil and apply to the palm of your hand, an oil inhaler, or a tissue. Bring the essential oils close to your nostrils and inhale the aroma deeply. You can cover one nostril at a time with your thumb and, if you prefer, alternate nostrils. This process sends the properties straight to your brain and the effects are immediate. You can complete this process 3–4 times daily.

Energizing Rub

Rub this on your neck, soles of your feet, or chest when you need the energy to accomplish that major task like painting a room or finishing a project. The essential oils in this recipe are all about energy and stamina due to their stimulating therapeutic properties. I usually make up a big bottle of this and rub it on every day till it's gone.

Yield: 1 fluid ounce

RECIPE
8 drops peppermint oil
7 drops lemon oil
5 drops eucalyptus oil
4 drops vitamin E oil
1 fluid ounce carrier oil

Pour the essential oils, carrier oil, and any remaining ingredients into a small glass container, bowl, or jar. Swirl or whisk to mix the ingredients and apply lightly to the area desired, such as pressure points, neck, soles of feet, temples, or chest. Keep essential oil mixture away from open wounds, mucus membranes, genitals, eyes, and sensitive areas. Repeat application as needed, usually 2–3 times daily. You may cover area with linen or cloth to protect clothing and furniture. Store unused portion in a glass jar or container with a tight-fitting lid in a cool, dark area for up to 3 months.

Wake Me in the Morning Bath

Some people like a "wake me up" bath in the morning, and some like a "calm me down" bath at night. This bath recipe is full of the essential oils that will most certainly wake you up and get your day started off right with their stimulating and energy-boosting properties.

Yield: 1 application

RECIPE

3 drops lemongrass oil

3 drops sage oil

3 drops fir oil

3 drops frankincense oil

1 drop eucalyptus oil

1 tablespoon carrier oil

1 tablespoon milk (optional for adults, recommended for children)

As you begin to fill the tub with water, pour the chosen essential oils and carrier oil into the running water. Run a warm, not hot, bath. Water that is too hot will cause the essential oils to dissipate. You may add 1 tablespoon of milk to the water; this ensures that the essential oils will not stick to your skin, but will mix with the water. You may soak in the water as long as you are comfortable. Dry your feet well once you get out of the water, as the oils will cause them to be slippery, increasing your chances of falling. Rinse the tub of any remaining oils.

Grounding

When a person is grounded, it means that emotionally, physically, spiritually, and mentally they are attached firmly to the earth. You are present in the here and now, without wandering thoughts, and able to focus and concentrate on the tasks at hand. Being grounded makes us readily available to our loved ones and makes us the type of person that others can count on. If you feel yourself unable to concentrate or are feeling scattered and foggy, you probably need a little grounding in your life.

Essential Oils

Benzoin, cedarwood, cypress, elemi, juniper, patchouli, rosewood, sandalwood, scots pine, spruce, and white fir

My Feet Are Roots

I personally love this foot rub. I often have issues with being grounded and have to surround myself with grounding colors, aromas, and therapeutic properties that I know will help me to focus and be present. When your thoughts feel flighty and you can't quite focus on any one particular thing, this blend will help you to have pinpoint focus and be more grounded.

Yield: 1 application

RECIPE
4 drops patchouli oil
4 drops elemi oil
2 drops vitamin E oil
1 teaspoon carrier oil

Pour the essential oils, carrier oil, and any remaining ingredients into a small glass container, bowl, or jar. Swirl or whisk to mix the ingredients and apply lightly to the area desired, such as pressure points, neck, soles of feet, temples, or chest. Keep essential oil mixture away from open wounds, mucus membranes, genitals, eyes, and sensitive areas. Repeat application as needed, usually 2–3 times daily. You may cover area with linen or cloth to protect clothing and furniture. Store unused portion in a glass jar or container with a tight-fitting lid in a cool, dark area for up to 3 months.

Grounding Laundry

Having your clothing constantly smell like grounding essential oils is a surefire way to help you become more firmly rooted to the earth. I absolutely love adding essential oils to my laundry detergent and it not only helps to clean my clothing, it diffuses the aromas throughout my home, and brings a lot of healing, peace, and contentment to me and my family.

Yield: 1 application

RECIPE

4 drops of any of the above mentioned essential oils for grounding

1 washer load amount of detergent

Pour the detergent needed into a small bowl. Add the essential oils to the detergent and use to wash laundry as usual.

Wet Ground Bath

When I notice that I am getting too flighty, talkative, impulsive, or ditzy, I realize that I need a good grounding bath. These essential oils in the bath not only smell heavenly, they bring me a sense of being rooted in the present and calm my soul.

Yield: 1 application

RECIPE

9 drops elemi oil

5 drops juniper oil

4 drops petitgrain oil

1 tablespoon milk (optional for adults, recommended for children)

As you begin to fill the tub with water, pour the chosen essential oils and carrier oil into the running water. Run a warm, not hot, bath. Water that is too hot will cause the essential oils to dissipate. You may add 1 tablespoon of milk to the water; this ensures that the essential oils will not stick to your skin, but will mix with the water. You may soak in the water as long as you are comfortable. Dry your feet well once you get out of the water, as the oils will cause them to be slippery, increasing your chances of falling. Rinse the tub of any remaining oils.

Grounding Lotion

The essential oils in this blend are chock-full of grounding essential oils. When you are feeling confused, flighty, and impulsive, this recipe works to balance you out and helps you to be at your best. This aroma works equally as well for men as women.

Yield: 1 fluid ounce

RECIPE

3 drops juniper oil

3 drops patchouli oil

2 drops rosewood oil

1 fluid ounce unscented body lotion

Add the recommended amount of essential oils to any brand of mild unscented lotion. Whisk until thoroughly mixed. Apply lotion to body as needed. Store unused portion in a jar with a tight-fitting lid in a cool, dark area for up to 3 months.

Intelligence

Increasing one's intelligence is one of the most sought-after paths taken by humans. Essential oils, these in particular, can cross that blood/brain barrier and work on expanding the pathway flow through the brain. These oils are known for preventing the breakdowns of the neurotransmitters. These blends and recipes have been utilized by many cultures over time to improve clarity, memory, and overall brain function, and heal brain diseases. The therapeutic properties that work here are analgesic, stimulant, nervine, tonic, and depurative properties, to name a few.

Essential Oils

Basil, clary sage, frankincense, juniper berry, lemon, mandarin, orange, peppermint, rosemary, sage, and tangerine

Brain Boost Spray

This recipe uses vital essential oils for giving your brain a boost of therapeutic properties that will increase the memory and help restore brain function. This is a great

222   CHAPTER 5

one to use before taking a test or heading out to that important meeting. Stimulating, tonic, and restorative properties help brains to function at their peak.

Yield: 2 fluid ounces

RECIPE
9 drops rosemary oil
6 drops peppermint oil
4 drops juniper berry oil
1 tablespoon witch hazel
2 fluid ounces water

Add all ingredients to a dark-colored spray bottle. Check for material steadfastness before spraying on fabric. Shake the bottle and spray onto area desired, such as body, hair, home, car, or office. Do not spray into or on open wounds, genitals, eyes, or mucus membranes. Store in a cool, dark area for up to 3 months. Shake well before each use to combine the ingredients.

Brain Circulatory Rub

This rub is great for applying to the temples to increase blood flow to the brain, enhance memory skills, and think much more clearly and precisely. If you have a problem and the answer eludes you, try this rub.

Yield: 1 tablespoon

RECIPE
3 drops clary sage oil
2 drops frankincense oil
2 drops basil oil
1 tablespoon carrier oil

Pour the essential oils, carrier oil, and any remaining ingredients into a small glass container, bowl, or jar. Swirl or whisk to mix the ingredients and apply lightly to the area desired, such as pressure points, neck, soles of feet, temples, or chest. Keep essential oil mixture away from open wounds, mucus membranes, genitals, eyes, and sensitive areas. Repeat application as needed, usually 2–3 times daily. You may cover area with linen or cloth to protect clothing and furniture. Store unused portion in a glass jar or container with a tight-fitting lid in a cool, dark area for up to 3 months.

Intelligence Bath

After the age of about seventy-five, the neurotransmitters in the brain get blocked and can't pass information from one part of the brain to another. These oils have been reported to help relieve some of those blockages and get the brain back on track. The brain-boosting properties in this blend include anti-inflammatory, restorative, stimulant, and tonic components.

Yield: 1 application

RECIPE
9 drops frankincense oil
5 drops rosemary oil
5 drops orange oil
1 tablespoon milk (optional for adults, recommended for children)
1 tablespoon carrier oil

As you begin to fill the tub with water, pour the chosen essential oils and carrier oil into the running water. Run a warm, not hot, bath. Water that is too hot will cause the essential oils to dissipate. You may add 1 tablespoon of milk to the water; this ensures that the essential oils will not stick to your skin, but will mix with the water. You may soak in the water as long as you are comfortable. Dry your feet well once you get out of the water, as the oils will cause them to be slippery, increasing your chances of falling. Rinse the tub of any remaining oils.

Citrus Brain Bombs

Citrus has been scientifically proven to increase brain performance. These three oils in particular out of the citrus oils have a good reputation for maximizing brain function. These are also the best-smelling bath bombs in the entire universe. You will fall in love with these aromas while improving your brain at the same time. Citrus contains anti-toxic agents to rid your body of heavy metals, increasing brain function.

Yield: 8–12 bombs

RECIPE
1 cup baking soda
½ cup citric acid
½ cup cornstarch
½ cup Epsom salts, fine grained
15 drops lemon oil
15 drops tangerine oil
5 drops mandarin oil
½ teaspoon carrier oil
¾ teaspoon water
spray bottle (water)

In a large bowl, mix your dry ingredients together until fine with a whisk. In a tiny jar with a lid, add your wet ingredients and shake to mix. You may add a couple drops of food coloring to the wet jar. Extremely slowly, add the wet ingredients to the dry ingredients while whisking rapidly. If fizzing takes place, whisk until it is mixed. Once the ingredients are well mixed, it should be the texture of slightly damp sand. Add a spray or two of water if needed. Once the mixture is the consistency you like, form into balls; I just smash mine down into ice cube trays or muffin tins. You can use cute molds, but you must work rapidly as mixture will dry out quickly. Leave in open air, uncovered, in a room where they will not be disturbed for 12–24 hours. Once they are dry, you can place 1–2 bombs into your bath or directly into the spray of the shower and they will fizz and release their aromatic and healing properties. Store unused portion in an airtight container for up to 6 months.

Intuition

Intuition is a gift that many of us are born with: the ability to just *know* when something is right or wrong. In order to hone your intuition skills, try one of the oils that have been used for thousands of years to sharpen that gut instinct. Many essential oils are reputed to heighten a person's skill and aid in the development of their intuition. Experiment with a few different recipes to find out which one gives you that intuitive edge.

Essential Oils

Clary sage, eucalyptus, frankincense, German chamomile, helichrysum, juniper, and patchouli

ESP Inhale

Many people are naturally open to their intuition, and some of us have to work at it. These essential oils have been used forever to open the mind, heart, and soul and receive the messages coming to us from the universe.

Yield: 1 application

RECIPE

1 drop clary sage oil

or

1 drop agrimony oil

or

1 drop patchouli oil

Choose your essential oil and apply to the palm of your hand, an oil inhaler, or a tissue. Bring the essential oils close to your nostrils and inhale the aroma deeply. You can cover one nostril at a time with your thumb and, if you prefer, alternate nostrils. This process sends the properties straight to your brain and the effects are immediate. You can complete this procedure 3–4 times daily.

Mind Reading Massage

These essential oils have been reported to allow us to connect fully with someone else, tune in to what they are feeling, and walk in their shoes with empathy through understanding. When you want to totally connect intuitively to another individual, this is the recipe for you.

Yield: 1 fluid ounce

RECIPE
7 drops frankincense oil
4 drops juniper oil
2 drops clary sage oil
1 fluid ounce carrier oil

Pour the essential oils and the carrier oil into a small glass container, bowl, or jar. Swirl to mix the ingredients and use to massage lightly the area desired, such as temples, neck, chest, back, or soles of feet. Keep essential oil mixture away from open wounds, mucus membranes, genitals, eyes, and sensitive areas. Repeat application as needed. Store unused portion in a glass jar or container with a tight-fitting lid in a cool, dark area for up to 3 months.

Spirit Spritzer

These essential oils are known to open the channels of communication between the spirits and us. Spray when you need spiritual help with answering a difficult question or choosing between options and cannot make that decision on your own.

Yield: 2 fluid ounces

RECIPE
9 drops German chamomile oil
5 drops frankincense oil
2 drops helichrysum oil
2 drops clary sage oil
1 tablespoon witch hazel
2 fluid ounces water

Spritzers are lighter than sprays, and easier to wear on the body or in your hair. Mix the essential oils, water, and witch hazel into a spray bottle. Shake well before each use. Lightly spray the area desired, such as body, hair, clothing (check first for color damage to clothing and furniture), rooms, car, or office. The lightly scented fragrance and the healing therapeutic properties will soon make this one of your favorite methods of using your oils. Store your spritzer in a cool, dark area for up to 3 months.

Connections Diffuser

This is a great diffuser recipe, long known to open passages between our intuition, our God, and us. When you have a period of time dedicated to meditation or prayer, this is the recipe you will cling to in times of needed connection.

Yield: 1 application

RECIPE
4 drops patchouli oil
4 drops juniper oil
3 drops helichrysum oil
2 drops eucalyptus oil
Water

Follow your directions for using essential oils in your particular brand of diffuser. Ensure that your diffuser does not use heat but runs by vibration, sound waves, or another cold-steam type of process. Choose the essential oils needed for your condition, then add water and oils to the diffuser. Run your diffuser as needed to permeate the air with therapeutic properties and achieve the results you desire.

Dreams Do Come True Powder

Some people feel that answers to difficult decisions or paths are given to them in their dreams. Multiply that exponentially when you use this nighttime powder under your sheets and sleep on it. The sedative properties along with the dream-inducing agents will have you intuitively coming to a decision by the time you wake up.

Yield: ½ cup

RECIPE
8 drops lavender oil
6 drops chamomile oil
3 drops frankincense oil

4 drops vitamin E oil

½ cup cornstarch

Place the ingredients into a mason jar, stirring well with a whisk. Carefully poke holes into the lid, use this as a shaker, and shake the ingredients into pillowcases or under sheet areas as needed. You can get a piece of plastic wrap and place it over the jar and under the lid to keep powder from spilling out when not in use. Store in a glass jar or container with a tight-fitting lid in a cool, dark, and dry area for up to 3 months.

Intuition Bath Salts

Relax in the tub with these mind-opening essential oils. Keep a pen and paper handy outside of the tub and write down whatever comes to your mind. Later, look at everything you have written and you may possibly find answers that you didn't even know you had within yourself.

Yield: 3 cups

RECIPE

5 drops juniper oil

5 drops clary sage oil

5 drops frankincense oil

3 drops helichrysum oil

5 drops vitamin E oil

3 cups salts

2 tablespoons carrier oil

1 tablespoon milk (optional for adults, recommended for children)

Use any type of salt you prefer: pink Himalayan salt, sea salt, Epsom salts, etc. In a small container, add the essential oils to the desired type of salt. Stir until well blended. Screw lid onto container tightly. Leave mixture in a dark area for 24 hours and then stir mixture again. Run the bathwater. Once the tub is full of water, you can add the milk, and then add ½ cup of the bath salt mixture to bathwater as you get into the tub. You may stay in the tub as long as the temperature is comfortable. Dry your feet well when you get out of the bath, as the oils are slippery and can cause you

to fall. Store remainder in a glass jar or container with a tight-fitting lid in a cool, dark area for up to 3 months. These jars make attractive, inexpensive, and healing gifts!

Love

Ahhh, who can live without love? Whether looking for the "right one" or spicing up the relationships we already have, essential oils are perfect for love and romance. Utilized for thousands of years by every culture from Native Americans to Egyptian princesses, the plants from which we extract these essential oils are said to have the solutions to our inquiries about love. There is an endless supply of recipes and potions to conjure up some love and romance in our lives.

Essential Oils

Basil, cardamom, cinnamon, coriander, frankincense, ginger, jasmine, lavender, lime, myrtle, peppermint, and rose

I Love You Massage

When these essential oils permeate the air, your loved one will know how much you treasure them when giving them this special massage with the aphrodisiacal properties inherent in this blend.

Yield: 1 fluid ounce

RECIPE
5 drops rose oil
5 drops jasmine oil
5 drops basil oil
5 drops lime oil
4 drops vitamin E oil
1 fluid ounce carrier oil

Pour the essential oils and the carrier oil into a small glass container, bowl, or jar. Swirl to mix the ingredients and use to massage lightly the area desired, such as temples, neck, chest, back, or soles of feet. Keep essential oil mixture away from open wounds, mucus membranes, genitals, eyes, and sensitive areas. Repeat application as needed. Store unused portion in a glass jar or container with a tight-fitting lid in a cool, dark area for up to 3 months.

Love Diffuser

This blend imparts an aroma into the air that invigorates certain hormones and pheromones due to aphrodisiacal properties. When you want a little extra help in the love department, this is a recipe that is sure to become one of your favorites.

Yield: 1 application

RECIPE
3 drops cardamom oil
2 drops cinnamon oil
2 drops peppermint oil
4 drops lavender oil
Water

Follow your directions for using essential oils in your particular brand of diffuser. Ensure that your diffuser does not use heat but runs by vibration, sound waves, or another cold-steam type of process. Choose the essential oils needed for your condition, then add water and oils to the diffuser. Run your diffuser as needed to permeate the air with therapeutic properties and achieve the results you desire.

Love Bath

These essential oils are reputed to have some of the most astounding aphrodisiacal qualities known. Run this in the bath (but preferably not when you're alone) to make romance a number one priority.

Yield: 1 application

RECIPE
6 drops rose oil
3 drops frankincense oil
4 drops myrtle oil

4 drops coriander oil

1 tablespoon carrier oil

1 tablespoon milk (optional)

As you begin to fill the tub with water, pour the chosen essential oils and carrier oil into the running water. Run a warm, not hot, bath. Water that is too hot will cause the essential oils to dissipate. You may add 1 tablespoon of milk to the water; this ensures that the essential oils will not stick to your skin, but will mix with the water. You may soak in the water as long as you are comfortable. Dry your feet well once you get out of the water, as the oils will cause them to be slippery, increasing your chances of falling. Rinse the tub of any remaining oils.

Spraying for Romance

Spray this blend when you want to catch the eye of that special someone and they won't pay attention. This spray is sure to inspire thoughts of love in anyone in the vicinity of these enticing aromas. These essential oils have been used for many years to bring about the one of one's life with the aphrodisiacal properties inherent in these oils.

Yield: 2 fluid ounces

RECIPE

2 drops clove oil

7 drops jasmine oil

4 drops lavender oil

3 drops cinnamon oil

1 tablespoon witch hazel

2 fluid ounces water

Add all ingredients to a dark-colored spray bottle. Check for material steadfastness before spraying on fabric. Shake the bottle and spray onto area desired, such as body, hair, home, car, or office. Do not spray into or on open wounds, genitals, eyes, or mucus membranes. Store in a cool, dark area for up to 3 months. Shake well before each use to combine the ingredients.

Love Linen Powder

Sprinkle this concoction under the linen to bring a little romance to your nights. Each of these oils is well known for their aphrodisiacal properties. This blend will help you acquire that much sought-after night of romance and love.

Yield: ½ cup

RECIPE
7 drops lavender oil
7 drops rose oil
7 drops jasmine oil
½ cup cornstarch
5 drops vitamin E oil

Place the ingredients into a mason jar, stirring well with a whisk. Carefully poke holes into the lid, use this as a shaker, and shake the ingredients into pillowcases or under sheet areas as needed. You can get a piece of plastic wrap and place it over the jar and under the lid to keep powder from spilling out when not in use. Store in a glass jar or container with a tight-fitting lid in a cool, dark, and dry area for up to 3 months.

Amour Bath Salts

These essential oils bring out the romantic side of people. Enjoy soaking in a tub of these beautiful aromas and bathing yourself in essential oils reputed to increase desire and romance.

Yield: 3 cups

RECIPE
7 drops cardamom oil
7 drops frankincense oil
7 drops myrtle oil
2 tablespoons carrier oil
5 drops vitamin E oil
3 cups salts
1 tablespoon milk (optional for adults)

Use any type of salt you prefer: pink Himalayan salt, sea salt, Epsom salts, etc. In a small container, add the essential oils to the desired type of salt. Stir until well blended. Screw lid onto container tightly. Leave mixture in a dark area for 24 hours and then stir mixture again. Run the bathwater. Once the tub is full of water, you can add the milk, and then add ½ cup of the bath salt mixture to bathwater as you get into the tub. You may stay in the tub as long as the temperature is comfortable. Dry your feet well when you get out of the bath, as the oils are slippery and can cause you to fall. Store remainder in a glass jar or container with a tight-fitting lid in a cool, dark area for up to 3 months. These jars make attractive, inexpensive, and healing gifts!

Memory

You can most surely count on forgetting information as you get older. Age is one of the most prevalent reasons for a person to have trouble with remembering things, especially more recent events. Most people have heard the saying that peppermint oil can help you to remember information when cramming for a test, but there are many more essential oils that you can use daily to stimulate the memory section of the brain. Oftentimes memory loss can also be associated with various illnesses, injuries, or life events so if memory loss is unbridled, it's best to have it checked out by a physician. Essential oils have been used for an eternity to help promote long- and short-term memory skills.

Essential Oils

Basil, cajeput, citrus, clary sage, frankincense, ginkgo biloba, lavender, lemon, lemongrass, melissa, orange, patchouli, peppermint, rosemary, vetiver, and white fir

Gentle Wind Powder

Strengthen your memory skills by sleeping on these essential oils known for their memory promoting elements. These oils will reportedly seep into the memory portion of your brain so you can wake up sharper, more focused, and able to recall needed details.

Yield: ¼ cup

RECIPE
3 drops melissa oil
3 drops rosemary oil
3 drops patchouli oil
4 drops vitamin E oil
¼ cup cornstarch

Place the ingredients into a mason jar, stirring well with a whisk. Carefully poke holes into the lid, use this as a shaker, and shake the ingredients into pillowcases or under sheet areas as needed. You can get a piece of plastic wrap and place it over the jar and under the lid to keep powder from spilling out when not in use. Store in a glass jar or container with a tight-fitting lid in a cool, dark, and dry area for up to 3 months.

Perfect Storm Bath Salts

Relax in the tub while these amazing essential oils increase your memory skills while at the same time imparting healing and aromatic benefits. More and more scientific research is becoming available to the public about how essential oils work wonders in healing memory issues in adults.

Yield: 3 cups

RECIPE
7 drops clary sage oil
7 drops cajeput oil
7 drops orange oil
2 tablespoons carrier oil
3 cups salts

Use any type of salt you prefer: pink Himalayan salt, sea salt, Epsom salts, etc. In a small container, add the essential oils to the desired type of salt. Stir until well blended. Screw lid onto container tightly. Leave mixture in a dark area for 24 hours and then stir mixture again. Run the bathwater. Once the tub is full of water, you can add the milk, and then add ½ cup of the bath salt mixture to bathwater as you get into the tub. You may stay in the tub as long as the temperature is comfortable. Dry your feet well when you get out of the bath, as the oils are slippery and can cause you to fall. Store remainder in a glass jar or container with a tight-fitting lid in a cool, dark area for up to 3 months. These jars make attractive, inexpensive, and healing gifts!

Zen Temple Rub

This recipe is great to use when you are going to take a test or for studying. These essential oils are well known for their memory-enhancing benefits.

Yield: 1 application

RECIPE
1 drop frankincense oil

or

1 drop peppermint oil

Combine the ingredients into a small bottle, bowl, or jar. This recipe uses the direct application process whereby you can apply drops of the blend to the temples. Do not apply directly to eyes, genitals, open wounds, or mucus membranes. Store in a bottle or glass jar or a container with a tight-fitting lid in a cool, dark area for up to 3 months.

Pleasant Memories Rub

Use these essential oils every day to assist in increasing your memory skills, while, at the same time, enjoying their healing benefits and pleasing aroma.

Yield: 1 fluid ounce

RECIPE
1 drop frankincense oil
1 drop patchouli oil
1 drop sandalwood oil
3 drops lemon oil
3 drops rosemary oil
3 drops vitamin E oil
1 fluid ounce carrier oil

Pour the essential oils, carrier oil, and any remaining ingredients into a small glass container, bowl, or jar. Swirl or whisk to mix the ingredients and apply lightly to the area desired, such as pressure points, neck, soles of feet, temples or chest. Keep essential oil mixture away from open wounds, mucus membranes, genitals, eyes, and sensitive areas. Repeat application as needed, usually 2–3 times daily. You may cover area with linen or cloth to protect clothing and furniture. Store unused portion in a glass jar or container with a tight-fitting lid in a cool, dark area for up to 3 months.

Air of Remembrance

Run this diffuser recipe to get the most benefits from these memory-invoking essential oils. Scientific studies have proven that aromas provoke the memory more than anything else.

Yield: 1 application

RECIPE
5 drops frankincense oil
3 drops lemongrass oil
3 drops peppermint oil
Water

Follow your directions for using essential oils in your particular brand of diffuser. Ensure that your diffuser does not use heat but runs by vibration, sound waves, or another cold-steam type of process. Choose the essential oils needed for your condition, then add water and oils to the diffuser. Run your diffuser as needed to permeate the air with therapeutic properties and achieve the results you desire.

Gentle Nudge Inhale

Use for a quick memory boost when you are about to undertake a challenge in which you feel the need to positively reinforce your memory skills.

Yield: 1 application

RECIPE
1 drop orange oil

or

1 drop cajeput oil

Choose your essential oil and apply to the palm of your hand, an oil inhaler, or a tissue. Bring the essential oils close to your nostrils and inhale the aroma deeply. You can cover one nostril at a time with your thumb and, if you prefer, alternate nostrils. This process sends the properties straight to your brain and the effects are immediate. You can complete this procedure 3–4 times daily.

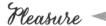

Pleasure

Pleasure is the state of the brain that provides you with happiness, contentment, joy, and overall good feelings. Finding pleasure in things is sometimes a matter of perception. While one person thinks that a walk in the woods is hot, tiresome, and annoying, another person may think it is very pleasurable. Finding pleasure can be as easy as thinking positively. These essential oils have been used for thousands of years to open the pleasure centers in our brains.

Essential Oils
Frankincense, juniper, melissa, myrrh, neroli, rose, and yarrow

Pagan's Aroma
Having this aroma drift throughout your home or office can bring a lot of pleasure to those fortunate enough to be in the vicinity. These essential oils bring pleasing memories and positive attitudes to the surface.

Yield: 1 application

RECIPE
5 drops neroli oil
5 drops juniper oil
Water

Follow your directions for using essential oils in your particular brand of diffuser. Ensure that your diffuser does not use heat but runs by vibration, sound waves, or another cold-steam type of process. Choose the essential oils needed for your condition, then add water and oils to the diffuser. Run your diffuser as needed to permeate the air with therapeutic properties and achieve the results you desire.

Heavenly Hands

This hand rub is quick and effective at bringing pleasurable feelings to your mind, body, and soul. I love to have this handy on those days that I am feeling anxious or down. I just dip my fingers in, rub, and inhale!

Yield: 1 tablespoon

RECIPE

3 drops rose oil

3 drops melissa oil

1 tablespoon grape seed oil

Combine the ingredients together into a small bowl. Dip one hand into the bowl until fingers are covered in the oils. Rub hands together for 5 minutes, rinse and repeat as needed. Ensure that the oils have been completely absorbed into your skin before touching furniture, clothing, etc., or oils will stain. You may pour remainder into a jar with a tight-fitting lid in a cool, dark area for up to 1 month.

Spiritual Exalting Inhale

Sometimes, simply inhaling an aroma from essential oils can bring immense pleasure. Just take a whiff of this the next time you are down and see if your spirits lift a little.

Yield: 1 application

RECIPE

1 drop frankincense oil

Choose your essential oil and apply to the palm of your hand, an oil inhaler, or a tissue. Bring the essential oils close to your nostrils and inhale the aroma deeply. You can cover one nostril at a time with your thumb and, if you prefer, alternate nostrils. This process sends the properties straight to your brain and the effects are immediate. You can complete this procedure 3–4 times daily.

Pleasurable Lotion

This lotion has the essential oils that were used by kings and queens to induce pleasurable emotions when they desired. Now you can have the same thing because this easily-made recipe uses essential oils that are readily available to bring pleasure and joy whenever you rub it in.

Yield: 1 fluid ounce

RECIPE
3 drops melissa oil
3 drops juniper oil
2 drops frankincense oil
1 fluid ounce unscented body lotion

Add the recommended amount of essential oils to any brand of mild unscented lotion. Whisk until thoroughly mixed. Apply lotion to body as needed. Store unused portion in a jar with a tight-fitting lid in a cool, dark area for up to 3 months.

Protection

Protection is a sense of safety and security from outside negative or evil influences. Essential oils (or the plants they have derived from) have been used for thousands of years to protect people from evil and negativity. People often use essential oils to meditate, pray, and to generally keep their souls safe while they open their hearts and minds to another plane of existence.

Essential Oils

Angelica, anise, benzoin, cedarwood, clove, cypress, dill, frankincense, fennel, hyssop, lavender, myrrh, petitgrain, rose, rosemary, vetiver, white birch, and ylang-ylang

Positivity Powder

This recipe includes essential oils known for their uplifting and positivity-inducing properties. Sprinkle this under all the sheets in the household to bring contentment, protection, and joy to everyone.

Yield: ¼ cup

RECIPE

5 drops angelica oil

3 drops lavender oil

3 drops frankincense oil

4 drops vitamin E oil

¼ cup cornstarch

Place the ingredients into a mason jar, stirring well with a whisk (the angelica oil is very thick, so whisk it well). Carefully poke holes into the lid, use this as a shaker, and shake the ingredients into pillowcases or under sheet areas as needed. You can get a piece of plastic wrap and place it over the jar and under the lid to keep powder from spilling out when not in use. Store in a glass jar or container with a tight-fitting lid in a cool, dark, and dry area for up to 3 months.

Protection Bath Salts

Feeling safe and secure is of utmost importance to most people. The essential oils used in this recipe have all been reported to bring safety and security to our environment. Using this bath recipe will help to protect you from evil, harm, and negativity.

Yield: 3 cups

RECIPE

5 drops cypress oil

5 drops hyssop oil

5 drops angelica oil

5 drops anise oil

5 drops vitamin E oil

2 tablespoons carrier oil

3 cups salts

1 tablespoon milk (optional for adults, recommended for children)

Use any type of salt you prefer: pink Himalayan salt, sea salt, Epsom salts, etc. In a small container, add the essential oils to the desired type of salt. Stir until well blended. Screw lid onto container tightly. Leave mixture in a dark area for 24 hours and then stir mixture again. Run the bathwater. Once the tub is full of water, you can add the milk, and then add ½ cup of the bath salt mixture to bathwater as you get into the tub. You may stay in the tub as long as the temperature is comfortable. Dry your feet well when you get out of the bath, as the oils are slippery and can cause you to fall. Store remainder in a glass jar or container with a tight-fitting lid in a cool, dark area for up to 3 months. These jars make attractive, inexpensive, and healing gifts!

Surrounded by Angels

This powerful recipe has been used forever and is reported to have the essential oils in it that will bring an army of angels to surround you and protect you from evil. This is a powerful blend of protective and peace-inducing oils that is ready in a spray bottle for you to use when you need it in a hurry. Just remember to shake well before using, as some of these oils are very thick, and the oils and water will separate after sitting.

Yield: 2 fluid ounces

RECIPE
3 drops agrimony oil
4 drops fennel oil
3 drops angelica oil
2 drops petitgrain oil
2 drops hyssop oil
1 tablespoon witch hazel
2 fluid ounces water

Add all ingredients to a dark-colored spray bottle. Check for material steadfastness before spraying on fabric. Shake the bottle and spray onto area desired, such as body, hair, home, car, or office. Do not spray into or on open wounds, genitals, eyes, or mucus membranes. Store in a cool, dark area for up to 3 months. Shake well before each use to combine the ingredients.

Force Field Air

These essential oils have long been reputed to protect you with a force field effect around your heart, home, family, and soul. Bring safety and security to all who are in the vicinity of this diffuser recipe. Use this recipe and help to keep those unwanted forces away!

Yield: 1 application

RECIPE
3 drops cypress oil
3 drops lime oil
3 drops rose oil
2 drops rosemary oil
Water

Follow your directions for using essential oils in your particular brand of diffuser. Ensure that your diffuser does not use heat but runs by vibration, sound waves, or another cold-steam type of process. Choose the essential oils needed for your condition, then add water and oils to the diffuser. Run your diffuser as needed to permeate the air with therapeutic properties and achieve the results you desire.

Instant Protection Inhaler

When I am feeling like I need an added boost of positivity and protection, this is my go-to recipe.

Yield: 1 application

RECIPE
1 drop angelica oil
or
1 drop myrrh oil
or
1 drop frankincense oil

Choose your essential oil and apply to the palm of your hand, an oil inhaler, or a tissue. Bring the essential oils close to your nostrils and inhale the aroma deeply. You can cover one nostril at a time with your thumb and, if you prefer, alternate nostrils. This process sends the properties straight to your brain and the effects are immediate. You can complete this procedure 3–4 times daily.

Echoes Drifting Bath

Take this bath and cover yourself with these protecting essential oils. Outside influences are said to be unable to penetrate the barrier created by these oils.

Yield: 1 application

RECIPE
5 drops rose oil
5 drops hyssop oil
5 drops ylang-ylang oil
1 tablespoon carrier oil
1 tablespoon milk (optional for adults, recommended for children)

As you begin to fill the tub with water, pour the chosen essential oils and carrier oil into the running water. Run a warm, not hot, bath. Water that is too hot will cause the essential oils to dissipate. You may add 1 tablespoon of milk to the water; this ensures that the essential oils will not stick to your skin, but will mix with the water. You may soak in the water as long as you are comfortable. Dry your feet well once you get out of the water, as the oils will cause them to be slippery, increasing your chances of falling. Rinse the tub of any remaining oils.

Security

Security is a feeling of safety, protection, and the absence of threat or fear. Sometimes, even if we are secure in our homes with our loved ones, we feel like we are unsafe. Illness, generalized anxiety, or even watching the news can provoke these feelings. These essential oils help to increase our feelings of safety and security with their calming and joyful properties.

Essential Oils

Angelica, cedarwood, frankincense, juniper berry, linden blossom, myrrh, patchouli, pine, spikenard, spruce, vetiver, white fir, and ylang-ylang

Simply Safe Bath

The essential oils in this bath are warming and relaxing. Becoming more grounded can help us to think clearly, feel a greater connection to family, and work on solving the problems before us. The anti-anxiety properties in this blend work together to help us feel more secure in ourselves and in the world around us.

Yield: 1 application

RECIPE
4 drops spikenard oil
4 drops linden blossom oil
4 drops juniper berry oil
1 tablespoon milk (optional for adults, recommended for children)
1 tablespoon carrier oil

As you begin to fill the tub with water, pour the chosen essential oils and carrier oil into the running water. Run a warm, not hot, bath. Water that is too hot will cause the essential oils to dissipate. You may add 1 tablespoon of milk to the water; this ensures that the essential oils will not stick to your skin, but will mix with the water. You may soak in the water as long as you are comfortable. Dry your feet well once you get out of the water, as the oils will cause them to be slippery, increasing your chances of falling. Rinse the tub of any remaining oils.

I'm a Force Spray

This is a great bedroom spray for anyone who is anxious or feeling unsafe. These properties will help to calm and ground them and let them know that they are okay, while at the same time promoting a good night's sleep.

Yield: 2 fluid ounces

RECIPE
5 drops pine oil
5 drops patchouli oil
5 drops myrrh oil
2 fluid ounces water
1 tablespoon witch hazel

Add all ingredients to a dark-colored spray bottle. Check for material steadfastness before spraying on fabric. Shake the bottle and spray onto area desired, such as body, hair, home, car, or office. Do not spray into or on open wounds, genitals, eyes, or mucus membranes. Store in a cool, dark area for up to 3 months. Shake well before each use to combine the ingredients.

Sleeping Safely Powder

This powder imparts a sense of relief, peace, calm, and security all night long. I use this in the guest room when I know I have company coming to spend the night and I want them to experience an ambiance of safety and security. They always remark how they slept like a baby!

Yield: ¼ cup

Recipe

8 drops vetiver oil

7 drops frankincense oil

6 drops angelica oil

4 drops vitamin E oil

¼ cup cornstarch

Place the ingredients into a mason jar, stirring well with a whisk. Carefully poke holes into the lid, use this as a shaker, and shake the ingredients into pillowcases or under sheet areas as needed. You can get a piece of plastic wrap and place it over the jar and under the lid to keep powder from spilling out when not in use. Store in a glass jar or container with a tight-fitting lid in a cool, dark, and dry area for up to 3 months.

Protective Shield

This blend helps the wearer to feel a shield of protection. These essential oils bring a sense of calm and relief, dispelling anxiety and worry. This roller bottle is handy to carry in your car or purse so that when you are feeling the need, it can be put on in moments.

Recipe

3 drops frankincense oil

3 drops juniper berry oil

3 drops ylang-ylang oil

2 drops vitamin E oil

1 fluid ounce carrier oil

Place the ingredients into a roller bottle. Roll around the area desired, such as wrist, neck, temples, soles of feet, or chest. Do not apply to open wounds, mucus membranes, eyes, or sensitive areas. Shake well before each use. Store unused portion in a glass jar or container with a tight-fitting lid in a cool, dark area for up to 3 months.

CHAPTER 6

Recipes for Desires

*E*veryone has desires for themselves and their loved ones. Desires are hopes and dreams of what we think will make our lives happier, fuller, and easier. These recipes have each been used for hundreds or thousands of years to help people obtain that which they passionately desire.

Abundance

Abundance is something that we all pray for, whether it is an abundance of love, money, health, respect, career goals, or a million other desires. Certain oils and fragrances have been used throughout time to help bring abundance into our personal existence. These oils have religious and holy significance in many cultures. For thousands of years, they have also been used to bring an abundance of positivity into a person's life and to eliminate all negativity. These oils boost good health for the immune system, lift the spirits, and diminish feelings of low self-esteem. Try them yourself to see if you can achieve an abundance of that which you desire.

Essential Oils

Black pepper, cedarwood, cinnamon bark, cinnamon leaf, clove, orange, and ylang-ylang

Abundance Bath Bombs

These bath and shower bombs have the tranquilizing, sedative, antirheumatic, antispasmodic, and tonic therapeutic properties needed to bring you to a place of ease, comfort, and enjoyment. These fizzy little pieces of heaven can help you to relax and open your heart to receive that which you ask for. Make these little treasures as gifts for those you wish to have an abundance of good in their lives. Bath bombs are inexpensive to make yourself and can bring you a world of positivity and goodness.

Yield: 12–18 bombs

RECIPE

1 cup baking soda

½ cup citric acid

½ cup cornstarch

½ cup Epsom salts, fine grained

15 drops orange oil

15 drops ylang-ylang oil

½ teaspoon carrier oil

¾ teaspoon water

spray bottle (water)

4 drops food coloring (optional)

In a large bowl, mix your dry ingredients together until fine with a whisk. In a tiny jar with a lid, add your wet ingredients and shake to mix. You may add a couple drops of food coloring to the wet jar. Extremely slowly, add the wet ingredients to the dry ingredients while whisking rapidly. If fizzing takes place, whisk until it is mixed. Once the ingredients are well mixed—it should be the texture of slightly damp sand—add a spray or two of water. Once the mixture is the consistency you like, form into balls; I just smash mine down into ice cube trays or muffin tins. You can use cute molds, but you must work rapidly as mixture will dry out quickly. Leave in open air, uncovered, in a room where they will not be disturbed for 12–24 hours. Once they are dry, you can place 1–2 bombs into your bath or directly into the spray of the shower and they will fizz and release their aromatic and healing properties. Store unused portion in an airtight container for up to 6 months.

Abundance Prayer

When spending time alone with your thoughts and prayers, it's optimal to have these essential oils permeating the air to help calm you, focus your thoughts, and bring peace to you and your household. The sedative, aphrodisiacal, antidepressant, nervine, and euphoric properties make this blend the optimal choice for prayer and meditation. This recipe is an all-time favorite to get that aroma diffusing around you as you seek abundance with your prayers of gratitude for all that you have yet to receive.

Yield: 1 application

RECIPE
3 drops ylang-ylang oil
3 drops frankincense oil
Water

Follow your directions for using essential oils in your particular brand of diffuser. Ensure that your diffuser does not use heat but runs by vibration, sound waves, or another cold-steam type of process. Choose the essential oils needed for your condition, then add water and oils to the diffuser. Run your diffuser as needed to permeate the air with therapeutic properties and achieve the results you desire.

Acquiring Oil

The aroma brought about by this recipe brings abundance and joy to the wearer. I like to wear this blend on the soles of my feet when I know I am going out to hunt for berries or herbs in the wild. I am then sure to bring back more than I thought I would and have plenty of an abundance left over to share with others. The therapeutic properties in this blend that give you the energy and strength you need for your projects are tonic, stimulant, and revitalizing agents.

Yield: 1 fluid ounce

RECIPE
1 fluid ounce carrier oil
7 drops sweet orange oil
6 drops myrrh oil

Combine the ingredients into a small bottle, bowl, or jar. This recipe uses the direct application process whereby you can apply drops of the blend to the soles of your feet, your neck, or anywhere you feel you would benefit. Do not apply directly to eyes, genitals, open wounds, or mucus membranes. Store in a bottle or glass jar or a container with a tight-fitting lid in a cool, dark area for up to 3 months.

Abundance Roll-On

Cover yourself with this blend that is believed to lead to an abundance of whatever you desire. These essential oils have been used for centuries to bring abundance to the wearer. This blend helps the wearer to feel a shield of protection. These essential oils bring a sense of calm and relief, dispelling anxiety and worry. This roller bottle is handy to carry in your car or purse so that when you are feeling the need, it can be put on in moments.

RECIPE
3 drops cedarwood oil
3 drops orange oil
3 drops ylang-ylang oil
2 drops vitamin E oil
1 fluid ounce carrier oil

Place the ingredients into a roller bottle. Roll around the area desired, such as wrist, neck, temples, soles of feet, or chest. Do not apply to open wounds, mucus membranes, eyes, or sensitive areas. Shake well before each use. Store unused portion in a glass jar or container with a tight-fitting lid in a cool, dark area for up to 3 months.

Answers (Divinations)

The recipes here are believed by many to open one up to receiving answers from the divine. These recipes are used primarily for prayer and meditation. Essential oils and the plants from which they derive have been used for thousands of years in rituals performed to receive answers from a higher power. Now you, too, can get answers to those questions that have plagued you forever while receiving the benefits of the therapeutic properties infused in these recipes.

Essential Oils

Agrimony, amber, angelica, basil, bay, camphor, carrot seed, clove, eucalyptus, fennel, frankincense, German chamomile, ginger, juniper, melissa, rosemary, sandalwood, and yarrow

Sleep On It Powder

The answers you seek will come more easily with this bedtime powder. Silently ponder on the question as you drift off to sleep. Then, when you awaken, your answer will be obvious, according to legends about this recipe. These oils contain nervine, tonic, sedative, analgesic, and calming properties.

Yield: ¼ cup

RECIPES
3 drops agrimony oil
3 drops angelica oil
3 drops frankincense oil
¼ cup cornstarch
4 drops vitamin E oil

Place the ingredients into a mason jar, stirring well with a whisk. Carefully poke holes into the lid, use this as a shaker, and shake the ingredients into pillowcases or under sheet areas as needed. You can get a piece of plastic wrap and place it over the jar and

under the lid to keep powder from spilling out when not in use. Store in a glass jar or container with a tight-fitting lid in a cool, dark, and dry area for up to 3 months.

I See Clearly Now Bath Salts

As you relax your mind and body with this soothing recipe, the answers you seek will just make sense to you as you remain calm and assess the situation. After using these salts, you should have insight into what direction you should go. The powerful circulatory, stimulating, tonic, antidepressant, cordial, nervine, sedative, and sudorific properties will help you maintain well-being and peace while seeking your answers.

Yield: 3 cups

RECIPES
5 drops amber oil
5 drops melissa oil
5 drops yarrow oil
5 drops juniper oil
2 tablespoons carrier oil
3 cups salts
1 tablespoon milk (optional for adults, recommended for children)

Use any type of salt you prefer: pink Himalayan salt, sea salt, Epsom salts, etc. In a small container, add the essential oils to the desired type of salt. Stir until well blended. Screw lid onto container tightly. Leave mixture in a dark area for 24 hours and then stir mixture again. Run the bathwater. Once the tub is full of water, you can add the milk, and then add ½ cup of the bath salt mixture to bathwater as you get into the tub. These jars make attractive, inexpensive, and healing gifts! Store remainder in cool, dark area in a glass jar or container with a tight-fitting lid for up to 3 months.

Openness Spray

Use this spray to open your mind to accepting what Spirit is trying to tell you. Spray it on before having a difficult conversation, prayer, meditation, or when making a tough decision. This spray has worked for me many times in making the decision of choosing the right path to take. The calming, sedative, aphrodisiac, and nervine properties work well together to bring you to a place of peace, relaxation, and clearheadedness.

Yield: 4 fluid ounces

RECIPES
10 drops melissa oil
2 drops sandalwood oil
2 drops angelica oil
1 tablespoon witch hazel
4 fluid ounces water

Add all ingredients to a dark-colored spray bottle. Check for material steadfastness before spraying on fabric. Shake the bottle and spray onto area desired. Do not spray into or on open wounds, genitals, eyes, or mucus membranes. Store in a cool, dark area for up to 3 months. Shake well before each use to combine the ingredients.

Bathe My Mind

Relax in the tub but don't worry about the answer; the correct answer will come to you as you soak in these divination-enhancing essential oils. The calming and healing therapeutic properties will relax you as you let your mind drift. By the time you towel off, you will have a clearer understanding of which direction you should proceed in.

Yield: 1 application

RECIPE
3 drops juniper oil
3 drops frankincense oil
2 drops German chamomile oil
1 drop yarrow oil
1 drop sandalwood oil
1 tablespoon carrier oil
1 tablespoon milk (optional for adults, recommended for children)

As you begin to fill the tub with water, pour the chosen essential oils and carrier oil into the running water. Run a warm, not hot, bath. Water that is too hot will cause the essential oils to dissipate. You may add 1 tablespoon of milk to the water; this ensures that the essential oils will not stick to your skin, but will mix with the water. You may soak in the water as long as you are comfortable. Dry your feet well once you get out of the water, as the oils will cause them to be slippery, increasing your chances of falling. Rinse the tub of any remaining oils.

Divination Air

Run this recipe in your diffuser before you open your home to another soul to discuss a particularly difficult situation, especially if you want to be able to speak from your heart and to speak the truth. The right answers will not only fill your mind, but fill the mind, heart, and soul of the person you are communicating with. The therapeutic properties inherent in this blend include antidepressant, cordial, nervine, sedative, tonic, and sudorific components.

Yield: 1 application

RECIPE
1 drop eucalyptus oil
1 drop carrot seed oil
3 drops melissa oil
2 drops ginger oil
Water

Follow your directions for using essential oils in your particular brand of diffuser. Ensure that your diffuser does not use heat but runs by vibration, sound waves, or another cold-steam type of process. Choose the essential oils needed for your condition, then add water and oils to the diffuser. Run your diffuser as needed to permeate the air with therapeutic properties and achieve the results you desire.

Truth Rub

If you are trying to find the solution to a particular problem, this is the perfect rub that will reveal the just and true way. Just a dab on your temples or on the soles of your feet will fill you with calming and wisdom-invoking properties that will give you the answers needed for your difficult decisions and to uncover that elusive truth that you seek.

Yield: 2 fluid ounces

RECIPE
5 drops melissa oil
2 drops juniper oil
2 drops rosemary oil
2 drops amber oil
2 drops bay oil
2 fluid ounces carrier oil

Pour the essential oils, carrier oil, and any remaining ingredients into a small glass container, bowl, or jar. Swirl or whisk to mix the ingredients and apply lightly to the area desired, such as temples, chest, neck, or soles of feet. Keep essential oil mixture away from open wounds, mucus membranes, genitals, eyes, and sensitive areas. Repeat application as needed, usually 2–3 times daily. You may cover area with linen or cloth to protect clothing and furniture. Store unused portion in a glass jar or container with a tight-fitting lid in a cool, dark area for up to 3 months.

Mind Expanding Inhale

This essential oil has been known to be a quick way to open your mind and allow you to accept the truth. When faced with two tough choices, this mind-opening oil will help you to calmly assess the pros and cons of both sides of the situation. The nervine, sedative, and calming properties of melissa oil will allow you to focus on the issues at hand and calm your mind enough to allow you to expand your consciousness to come to the best conclusion for you.

Yield: 1 application

RECIPE
2 drops melissa oil

Choose your essential oil and apply to the palm of your hand, an oil inhaler, or a tissue. Bring the essential oils close to your nostrils and inhale the aroma deeply. You can

cover one nostril at a time with your thumb and, if you prefer, alternate nostrils. This process sends the properties straight to your brain and the effects are immediate. You can complete this process 3–4 times daily.

Aphrodisiac

An aphrodisiac is a substance used to increase sexual desire. There have been many fables and tales about food, fragrances, colors, and lighting used as aphrodisiacs in English literature. Essential oils, herbs, and flowers have been used throughout the ages to increase sexual appetite in others and in ourselves. There are a myriad of reasons, both mental and physical, why we lose our sexual desire. Aphrodisiacs can work wonders on increasing your desire for lovemaking, or you can increase the desire that others may have for you!

Essential Oils

Amber, cardamom, cinnamon, clary sage, coriander, ginseng, jasmine, neroli, patchouli, rose, sandalwood, vanilla, and ylang-ylang

Hot, Hot, Hot

This oil blend will turn your partner's thoughts to you and you alone. Essential oils are used, as they have been for centuries, to cast a spell of love with their aphrodisiac and euphoric therapeutic properties.

Yield: 1 fluid ounce

RECIPE
2 drops clary sage oil
2 drops jasmine oil
1 drop vanilla oil
2 drops ylang-ylang oil
3 drops vitamin E oil
1 tablespoon carrier oil

Pour the essential oils and the carrier oil into a small glass container, bowl, or jar. Swirl to mix the ingredients and use to massage lightly the area desired, such as temples, neck, chest, back, or soles of feet. Keep essential oil mixture away from open wounds, mucus membranes, genitals, eyes, and sensitive areas. Repeat application as needed. Store unused portion in a glass jar or container with a tight-fitting lid in a cool, dark area for up to 3 months.

Fragrant Love Diffuser

When setting the mood for love, this is the aroma that should be filling your home. The essential oil's heady, earthy aroma is sexuality and seduction at its finest. Aphrodisiac properties along with tonic and sedative qualities give this recipe its setting for love.

Yield: 1 application

RECIPE
1 drop sandalwood oil
1 drop neroli oil
1 drop cinnamon oil
1 drop amber oil
Water

Follow your directions for using essential oils in your particular brand of diffuser. Ensure that your diffuser does not use heat but runs by vibration, sound waves, or another cold-steam type of process. Choose the essential oils needed for your condition, then add water and oils to the diffuser. Run your diffuser as needed to permeate the air with therapeutic properties and achieve the results you desire.

Sexual Soak

This works best if your bath time is shared with your partner or someone you love. Soak into this blend of essential oils and be transported to a world of decadence and pleasure. The therapeutic aphrodisiacal properties awaken sexual feelings in our partners and ourselves.

Yield: 1 application

RECIPE
2 drops jasmine oil
1 drop ginseng oil
2 drops rose oil
1 drop sandalwood oil
1 drop coriander oil
1 tablespoon carrier oil
1 tablespoon milk

As you begin to fill the tub with water, pour the chosen essential oils and carrier oil into the running water. Run a warm, not hot, bath. Water that is too hot will cause the essential oils to dissipate. You may add 1 tablespoon of milk to the water; this ensures that the essential oils will not stick to your skin, but will mix with the water. You may soak in the water as long as you are comfortable. Dry your feet well once you get out of the water, as the oils will cause them to be slippery, increasing your chances of falling. Rinse the tub of any remaining oils. In this case, two persons soaking is even better!

Love Linen

Nighttime is the right time for love when you discreetly sprinkle this sensual powder between the sheets. These essential oils are difficult to take in without thinking of loving the one you're with. This recipe contains aphrodisiac, tonic, stimulating, and calming therapeutic compounds to help you and your partner find that groove you've been missing.

Yield: ¼ cup

RECIPE
4 drops rose oil
4 drops jasmine oil
4 drops patchouli oil
4 drops sandalwood oil

¼ cup cornstarch

4 drops vitamin E oil

Place the ingredients into a mason jar, stirring well with a whisk. Carefully poke holes into the lid, use this as a shaker, and shake the ingredients into pillowcases or under sheet areas as needed. You can get a piece of plastic wrap and place it over the jar and under the lid to keep powder from spilling out when not in use. Store in a glass jar or container with a tight-fitting lid in a cool, dark, and dry area for up to 3 months.

Sex in a Bottle

Watch your partner's thoughts turn from the outside world to you with this sexually enticing scent lingering in the air. The essential oils in this combination are otherwise known as "sex in a bottle." They contain such properties as aphrodisiac, nervine, and antidepressant components to arouse anybody, anywhere, anytime.

Yield: 2 fluid ounces

RECIPE

5 drops rose oil

5 drops jasmine oil

5 drops ylang-ylang oil

2 drops neroli oil

1 tablespoon witch hazel

2 fluid ounces water

Add all ingredients to a dark-colored spray bottle. Check for material steadfastness before spraying on fabric. Shake the bottle and spray onto area desired. Do not spray into or on open wounds, genitals, eyes, or mucus membranes. You can spray this in a room that you will be in with the one you hope to love, and they will also reap the benefits of these love-inducing oils. Store in a cool, dark area for up to 3 months. Shake well before each use to combine the ingredients.

Sexy Time Bath Salts

Bring the sexual experience to the bath with this desire-invoking recipe. The qualities contained in this blend include stimulant, aphrodisiac, and tonic therapeutic properties.

Yield: 3 cups

RECIPE
5 drops ginseng oil
5 drops vanilla oil
5 drops cardamom oil
2 tablespoons carrier oil
3 cups salts
1 tablespoon milk (optional for adults, recommended for children)

Use any type of salt you prefer: pink Himalayan salt, sea salt, Epsom salts, etc. In a small container, add the essential oils to the desired type of salt. Stir until well blended. Screw lid onto container tightly. Leave mixture in a dark area for 24 hours and then stir mixture again. Run the bathwater. Once the tub is full of water, you can add the milk, and then add ½ cup of the bath salt mixture to bathwater as you get into the tub. You may stay in the tub as long as the temperature is comfortable. Dry your feet well when you get out of the bath, as the oils are slippery and can cause you to fall. Store remainder in a glass jar or container with a tight-fitting lid in a cool, dark area for up to 3 months. These jars make attractive, inexpensive, and healing gifts!

Confidence

This is a general feeling of how people feel about themselves and how they may react or relate to the world around them. Confidence is something that we learn to have and display outwardly to others. We can learn to have confidence in our work, in our abilities, and in our relationships. You know those people who are so confident about themselves that they just exude charisma? You can be one of those people. There are essential oils reputed to assist a person with gaining confidence in himself or herself.

Essential Oils

Basil, bay laurel, benzoin, bergamot, cassia, cedarwood, cypress, frankincense, geranium, jasmine, melissa, orange, peppermint, sandalwood, vetiver, and ylang-ylang

I'm Worth It Linen Powder

Put this powder between the sheets so that when you wake up in the morning, you will have a brighter outlook on life in general, but you will also feel good about yourself.

Yield: ¼ cup

RECIPE

3 drops cypress oil
3 drops basil oil
3 drops jasmine oil
4 drops vitamin E oil
¼ cup cornstarch

Place the ingredients into a mason jar, stirring well with a whisk. Carefully poke holes into the lid, use this as a shaker, and shake the ingredients into pillowcases or under sheet areas as needed. You can get a piece of plastic wrap and place it over the jar and under the lid to keep powder from spilling out when not in use. Store in a glass jar or container with a tight-fitting lid in a cool, dark, and dry area for up to 3 months.

Confident Atmosphere Diffuser

This diffuser recipe will let you know that you are the bomb! You can amp up your self-esteem with the essential oils in this recipe responsible for its confidence-boosting aroma. Believe in yourself, your vision, and your needs.

Yield: 1 application

RECIPE

3 drops jasmine oil
2 drops melissa oil
2 drops vetiver oil
1 drop basil oil
Water

Follow your directions for using essential oils in your particular brand of diffuser. Ensure that your diffuser does not use heat but runs by vibration, sound waves, or an-

other cold-steam type of process. Choose the essential oils needed for your condition, then add water and oils to the diffuser. Run your diffuser as needed to permeate the air with therapeutic properties and achieve the results you desire.

I'm the Greatest and I Know It Rub

Going for an interview? Going on a first date? Rub a little of this essential oil power-packing recipe and you will have calm nerves, self-worth, and feel great! Rid yourself of any fears or anxiety and go into that scary place feeling that you can accomplish anything and come out on top.

Yield: 2 tablespoons

RECIPE
3 drops ylang-ylang oil
2 drops orange oil
2 drops frankincense oil
1 drop bergamot oil
3 drops vitamin E oil
2 tablespoons carrier oil

Pour the essential oils, carrier oil, and any remaining ingredients into a small glass container, bowl, or jar. Swirl or whisk to mix the ingredients and apply lightly to the area desired, such as pressure points, neck, soles of feet, temples, or chest. Keep essential oil mixture away from open wounds, mucus membranes, genitals, eyes, and sensitive areas. Repeat application as needed, usually 2–3 times daily. You may cover area with linen or cloth to protect clothing and furniture. Store unused portion in a glass jar or container with a tight-fitting lid in a cool, dark area for up to 3 months.

Poise Spray

Have things gone wrong in your life lately? Don't let them see you sweat! The essential oils in this spray will have you smiling with confidence and a sense of purpose. Carry this in your purse or car and use whenever you just need to gain that little boost of confidence that will let the way you carry yourself show others your self-worth.

Yield: 2 fluid ounces

RECIPE

5 drops peppermint oil

2 drops melissa oil

2 drops jasmine oil

3 drops vetiver oil

3 drops vitamin E oil

1 tablespoon witch hazel

2 fluid ounces water

Add all ingredients to a dark-colored spray bottle. Check for material steadfastness before spraying on fabric. Shake the bottle and spray onto area desired, such as body, hair, home, car, or office. Do not spray into or on open wounds, genitals, eyes, or mucus membranes. Store in a cool, dark area for up to 3 months. Shake well before each use to combine the ingredients.

Confidence-Boosting Bath Salts

These essential oils are reported to make people feel great about themselves. Relax in this bath and you will come out knowing that you are a unique and wonderful soul on this planet.

Yield: 3 cups

RECIPE

8 drops orange oil

5 drops melissa oil

5 drops bergamot oil

2 tablespoons carrier oil

4 drops vitamin E oil

3 cups salts

1 tablespoon milk (optional for adults, recommended for children)

Use any type of salt you prefer: pink Himalayan salt, sea salt, Epsom salts, etc. In a small container, add the essential oils to the desired type of salt. Stir until well blended. Screw lid onto container tightly. Leave mixture in a dark area for 24 hours and then stir mixture again. Run the bathwater. Once the tub is full of water, you can add the milk, and then add ½ cup of the bath salt mixture to bathwater as you get into the tub. You may stay in the tub as long as the temperature is comfortable. Dry your feet well when you get out of the bath, as the oils are slippery and can cause you to fall. Store remainder in a glass jar or container with a tight-fitting lid in a cool, dark area for up to 3 months. These jars make attractive, inexpensive, and healing gifts!

Creativity

Creativity is our delightful characteristic that allows us to make something from nothing using ideas, imagination, thought, and necessity. Oftentimes life, with all of its demands, gets in the way of our creativity and imagination. These essential oils are reputed to boost that part of the brain that gets those light bulbs going off, filling our heads with ideas. I am a very creative person and love to busy myself with an endless supply of projects. These oils assist me with ideas and energy to make something out of nothing on a regular basis, not to mention how great these oils smell.

Essential Oils

Bay laurel, geranium, helichrysum, neroli, orange, and patchouli

Creativity Linen Powder

This is a wonderful powder for boosting the creativity in any type of artist. Sprinkle this under your sheets, have a very pleasant night's sleep, and wake up with that one great idea you have been waiting for. Get your brain working for you while you sleep!

Yield: 10–20 applications

RECIPE
3 drops orange oil
3 drops neroli oil
3 drops bay laurel oil
4 drops vitamin E oil
¼ cup cornstarch

Place the ingredients into a mason jar, stirring well with a whisk. Carefully poke holes into the lid, use this as a shaker, and shake the ingredients into pillowcases or under sheet areas as needed. You can get a piece of plastic wrap and place it over the jar and under the lid to keep powder from spilling out when not in use. Store in a glass jar or container with a tight-fitting lid in a cool, dark, and dry area for up to 3 months.

Idea Inhale

These essential oils are perfect for when you need an idea and you need it now! Get those creative juices flowing again with a simple inhale of one of these essential oils reported to boost memory, focus, and attention to detail.

Yield: 1 application

RECIPE
1 drop helichrysum oil
or
1 drop orange oil

Choose your essential oil and apply to the palm of your hand, an oil inhaler, or a tissue. Bring the essential oils close to your nostrils and inhale the aroma deeply. You can cover one nostril at a time with your thumb and, if you prefer, alternate nostrils. This process sends the properties straight to your brain and the effects are immediate. You can complete this process 3–4 times daily.

Creative Juices Diffuser

Diffuse this recipe when you are trying to write that book, paint that masterpiece, or write that perfect bar of music. The creative juices will reportedly flow like magic.

Yield: 1 application

RECIPE
3 drops geranium oil
2 drops neroli oil
2 drops bay laurel oil
Water

Follow your directions for using essential oils in your particular brand of diffuser. Ensure that your diffuser does not use heat but runs by vibration, sound waves, or another cold-steam type of process. Choose the essential oils needed for your condition, then add water and oils to the diffuser. Run your diffuser as needed to permeate the air with therapeutic properties and achieve the results you desire.

Imagination Spray

You can carry this spray with you, leave one at the office, carry one in your car, and use it anytime you need to get those creative juices flowing. The plants that these essential oils were derived from have been used for centuries to bring creativity to an otherwise overworked mind. Be free with your ideas and let them out. The book I am writing, the computer I am typing on, the chair I am sitting in, and the music I am listening to all came about because someone had an idea. Let your idea be the beginning of your future.

Yield: 2 fluid ounces

RECIPE
3 drops orange oil
2 drops patchouli oil
2 drops helichrysum oil
3 drops vitamin E oil
1 tablespoon witch hazel
2 fluid ounces water

Add all ingredients to a dark-colored spray bottle. Check for material steadfastness before spraying on fabric. Shake the bottle and spray onto area desired, such as body, hair, home, car, or office. Do not spray into or on open wounds, genitals, eyes, or mucus membranes. Store in a cool, dark area for up to 3 months. Shake well before each use to combine the ingredients.

Thinking of Wonders Massage

Use this oil blend when getting a massage and the ideas will flow while you rest and have a wonderful, creative, dreamlike massage. These oils have been used forever to induce the imagination and light the spark of creativity.

Yield: 1–2 applications

RECIPE

3 drops patchouli oil

2 drops geranium oil

2 drops neroli oil

1 drop orange oil

3 drops vitamin E oil

1 tablespoon carrier oil

Pour the essential oils and the carrier oil into a small glass container, bowl, or jar. Swirl to mix the ingredients and use to massage lightly the area desired, such as temples, neck, chest, back, or soles of feet. Keep essential oil mixture away from open wounds, mucus membranes, genitals, eyes, and sensitive areas. Repeat application as needed. Store unused portion in a glass jar or container with a tight-fitting lid in a cool, dark area for up to 3 months.

Creativity Bath Salts

Close your eyes while resting in this bath and let the creative energy of these essential oils overtake you and bring your ideas to the forefront. Your plans will begin to form and you will find a way to do what you need to do. You can think outside of the box and create something new and totally you!

Yield: 3 cups

RECIPE

5 drops bay laurel oil

5 drops geranium oil

5 drops orange oil

2 tablespoons carrier oil

4 drops vitamin E oil

3 cups salts

1 tablespoon milk (optional for adults, recommended for children)

Use any type of salt you prefer: pink Himalayan salt, sea salt, Epsom salts, etc. In a small container, add the essential oils to the desired type of salt. Stir until well blended. Screw lid onto container tightly. Leave mixture in a dark area for 24 hours and then stir mixture again. Run the bathwater. Once the tub is full of water, you can add the milk, and then add ½ cup of the bath salt mixture to bathwater as you get into the tub. You may stay in the tub as long as the temperature is comfortable. Dry your feet well when you get out of the bath, as the oils are slippery and can cause you to fall. Store remainder in a glass jar or container with a tight-fitting lid in a cool, dark area for up to 3 months. These jars make attractive, inexpensive, and healing gifts!

Gratitude

I truly believe that one of the greatest lessons I was taught in my life was learning to have gratitude and be thankful for myself, my family, and a million other things. I am even grateful every day for things I haven't received yet, but know that I will, in time, and when the time is perfect. Essential oils, herbs, and other treasures have been implemented throughout the ages as offerings to help us express our gratitude, to use during prayers of thanks, and to give our wishes a vehicle of transport to the heavens. Be thankful, be grateful; it works.

Essential Oils

Bergamot, cedarwood, coriander, frankincense, myrrh, rose, scots pine, and ylang-ylang

Thank You Spray

This spray is the gratitude-inducing aroma I use when I'm about to embark on a prayer of thankfulness. This blend calms me, helps me to focus, and gives me a happy perspective on life.

Yield: 2 fluid ounces

RECIPE

16 drops rose oil

12 drops bergamot oil

· 1 tablespoon witch hazel

2 fluid ounces water

Add all ingredients to a dark-colored spray bottle. Check for material steadfastness before spraying on fabric. Shake the bottle and spray onto area desired, such as body, hair, home, car, or office. Do not spray into or on open wounds, genitals, eyes, or mucus membranes. Store in a cool, dark area for up to 3 months. Shake well before each use to combine the ingredients.

Gratitude Massage Oil

Getting a massage is a very good time to count your blessings, not only for the massage, but for all that which you have and all that which you wish to receive. These relaxing blends will help you to feel great while imparting a sense of calm and peace in order to help you to focus on your prayers of gratitude.

Yield: 1 application

RECIPE

8 drops ylang-ylang oil

6 drops cedarwood oil

4 drops vitamin E oil

2 tablespoons carrier oil

Pour the essential oils and the carrier oil into a small glass container, bowl, or jar. Swirl to mix the ingredients and use to massage lightly the area desired, such as temples, neck, chest, back, or soles of feet. Keep essential oil mixture away from open wounds, mucus membranes, genitals, eyes, and sensitive areas. Repeat application as needed. Store unused portion in a glass jar or container with a tight-fitting lid in a cool, dark area for up to 3 months.

I Am Blessed Bath Bombs

As you luxuriate in your bath, be thankful. As you smell the aromas of these oils that have been used in rituals for a millennium, be thankful. As you ponder the path of your soul, be thankful. As you think of the food you will prepare when you get through with your bath, be thankful. Above all else, be thankful.

Yield: 8–12 bombs

RECIPE

1 cup baking soda

½ cup citric acid

½ cup cornstarch

½ cup Epsom salts, fine grained

15 drops frankincense oil

15 drops myrrh oil

½ teaspoon carrier oil

¾ teaspoon water

spray bottle (water)

In a large bowl, mix your dry ingredients together until fine with a whisk. In a tiny jar with a lid, add your wet ingredients and shake to mix. You may add a couple drops of food coloring to the wet jar. Extremely slowly, add the wet ingredients to the dry ingredients while whisking rapidly. If fizzing takes place, whisk until it is mixed. Once the ingredients are well mixed, it should be the texture of slightly damp sand. Add a spray or two of water if needed. Once the mixture is the consistency you like, form into balls; I just smash mine down into ice cube trays or muffin tins. You can use cute molds, but you must work rapidly as mixture will dry out quickly. Leave in open air, uncovered, in a room where they will not be disturbed for 12–24 hours. Once they are dry, you can place 1–2 bombs into your bath or directly into the spray of the shower and they will fizz and release their aromatic and healing properties. Store unused portion in an airtight container for up to 6 months.

Gratitude Roll-On

This roll-on contains essential oils that help you to be thankful for what you have and what you want. Easy to make and carry, this blend contains essential oils that have been used for centuries in rituals of gratitude. These essential oils bring a sense of calm and relief, dispelling anxiety and worry. This roller bottle is handy to carry in your car or purse so that when you are feeling the need, it can be put on in moments.

RECIPE

3 drops rose oil

3 drops frankincense oil

3 drops myrrh oil

2 drops vitamin E oil

1 fluid ounce carrier oil

Place the ingredients into a roller bottle. Roll around the area desired, such as wrist, neck, temples, soles of feet, or chest. Do not apply to open wounds, mucus membranes, eyes, or sensitive areas. Shake well before each use. Store unused portion in a glass jar or container with a tight-fitting lid in a cool, dark area for up to 3 months.

Harmony

Whether one wishes to experience harmony with themselves or with others around them, there are essential oils that can assist you with obtaining harmony in your life. Harmony in one's relationships, career, home, spirituality, and family is something that is fleeting and should be worked on daily.

Essential Oils

Amber, angelica, frankincense, geranium, hyssop, lavender, lemon, orange, palmarosa, Roman chamomile, rose, sage, sandalwood, and spruce

Come Together Linen Powder

This blend of essential oils is reputed to bring peace and harmony to everyone they touch. Calming, aphrodisiac, and sedative properties work together to relax your spirit and help you with enjoying peace and harmony throughout the night.

Yield: ¼ cup

RECIPE

3 drops angelica oil

3 drops palmarosa oil

3 drops lavender oil

4 drops vitamin E oil

¼ cup cornstarch

Place the ingredients into a mason jar, stirring well with a whisk. Carefully poke holes into the lid, use this as a shaker, and shake the ingredients into pillowcases or under sheet areas as needed. You can get a piece of plastic wrap and place it over the jar and under the lid to keep powder from spilling out when not in use. Store in a glass jar or container with a tight-fitting lid in a cool, dark, and dry area for up to 3 months.

Harmony Bath Salts

This recipe is meant to be shared by two people. Come together with a harmonizing blend of essential oils that unite, uplift, and connect two people mentally and spiritually. This bath recipe will bring positive energy to both of you, and you can communicate and unite in ways that will be worth remembering.

Yield: 3 cups

RECIPE

7 drops Roman chamomile oil

7 drops angelica oil

7 drops sandalwood oil

2 tablespoons carrier oil

5 drops vitamin E oil

3 cups salts

1 tablespoon milk (optional for adults, recommended for children)

Use any type of salt you prefer: pink Himalayan salt, sea salt, Epsom salts, etc. In a small container, add the essential oils to the desired type of salt. Stir until well blended. Screw lid onto container tightly. Leave mixture in a dark area for 24 hours and then stir mixture again. Run the bathwater. Once the tub is full of water, you can add the milk, and then add ½ cup of the bath salt mixture to bathwater as you get into the tub. You may stay in the tub as long as the temperature is comfortable. Dry your feet well when you get out of the bath, as the oils are slippery and can cause you to fall. Store remainder in a glass jar or container with a tight-fitting lid in a cool, dark area for up to 3 months. These jars make attractive, inexpensive, and healing gifts!

I Love You Too Diffuser

A harmonized household is a peaceful household. When this diffuser recipe of essential oils runs, watch the joy, peace, and laughter spread throughout your home. Harmony in the home is sometimes a lifelong endeavor. This blend will help you to achieve that goal now.

Yield: 1 application

RECIPE

5 drops orange oil

3 drops rose oil

2 drops hyssop oil

2 drops palmarosa oil

Water

Follow your directions for using essential oils in your particular brand of diffuser. Ensure that your diffuser does not use heat but runs by vibration, sound waves, or another cold-steam type of process. Choose the essential oils needed for your condition, then add water and oils to the diffuser. Run your diffuser as needed to permeate the air with therapeutic properties and achieve the results you desire.

Together We Stand Massage

When facing a tough battle, it is better to show a united front. Massage each other with this blend and nothing can break you apart. Balancing and harmonizing properties will give you harmony within yourself and with your partner.

Yield: 1 fluid ounce

RECIPE

2 drops amber oil

2 drops orange oil

2 drops geranium oil

4 drops ylang-ylang oil

4 drops vitamin E oil

1 fluid ounce carrier oil

Pour the essential oils and the carrier oil into a small glass container, bowl, or jar. Swirl to mix the ingredients and use to massage lightly the area desired, such as temples, neck, chest, back, or soles of feet. Keep essential oil mixture away from open wounds, mucus membranes, genitals, eyes, and sensitive areas. Repeat application as needed. Store unused portion in a glass jar or container with a tight-fitting lid in a cool, dark area for up to 3 months.

Harmony Inhale

Using this inhale when feeling disconnected is a great way to calm and soothe your mind and will help you get back on track with those around you. These aphrodisiac, calming, and soothing properties will bring harmony and peace quickly.

Yield: 1 application

RECIPE

1 drop lavender oil

or

1 drop frankincense oil

Choose your essential oil and apply to the palm of your hand, an oil inhaler, or a tissue. Bring the essential oils close to your nostrils and inhale the aroma deeply. You can

cover one nostril at a time with your thumb and, if you prefer, alternate nostrils. This process sends the properties straight to your brain and the effects are immediate. You can complete this procedure 3–4 times daily.

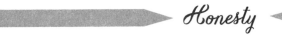

Honesty

There are essential oils reputed to bring out honesty in ourselves and in those around us. Oftentimes we are not honest with ourselves about how we feel about a particular dilemma, person, or situation in our lives. Applying essential oils to our surroundings and ourselves can assist us in answering those tough questions with a truthful answer that is often unknown, even to ourselves.

Essential Oils

Basil, cassia, citrus, cypress, frankincense, geranium, grapefruit, lemon, lime, melissa, orange, sandalwood, vetiver, and ylang-ylang

Honest with Myself Powder

When weighing the pros and cons of a painful decision, sleep on it with this honesty-invoking powder. This recipe is packed full of essential oils reputed to help a person with maintaining honesty in all situations. You will wake up and be truthful with yourself and give yourself the ability to forge ahead with your decision.

Yield: ¼ cup

RECIPE
3 drops geranium oil
3 drops lime oil
3 drops frankincense oil
4 drops vitamin E oil
¼ cup cornstarch

Place the ingredients into a mason jar, stirring well with a whisk. Carefully poke holes into the lid, use this as a shaker, and shake the ingredients into pillowcases or under sheet areas as needed. You can get a piece of plastic wrap and place it over the jar and

under the lid to keep powder from spilling out when not in use. Store in a glass jar or container with a tight-fitting lid in a cool, dark, and dry area for up to 3 months.

Truth-Telling Bath Salts

Take this bath with your partner and you can have the honest conversation that you have wanted and needed. The plants that these essential oils derive from have been used to get to the bottom of the truth for generations.

Yield: 3 cups

RECIPE

7 drops ylang-ylang oil

6 drops vetiver oil

5 drops orange oil

3 cups salts

5 drops vitamin E oil

2 tablespoons carrier oil

1 tablespoon milk (optional for adults, recommended for children)

Use any type of salt you prefer: pink Himalayan salt, sea salt, Epsom salts, etc. In a small container, add the essential oils to the desired type of salt. Stir until well blended. Screw lid onto container tightly. Leave mixture in a dark area for 24 hours and then stir mixture again. Run the bathwater. Once the tub is full of water, you can add the milk, and then add ½ cup of the bath salt mixture to bathwater as you get into the tub. You may stay in the tub as long as the temperature is comfortable. Dry your feet well when you get out of the bath, as the oils are slippery and can cause you to fall. Store remainder in a glass jar or container with a tight-fitting lid in a cool, dark area for up to 3 months. These jars make attractive, inexpensive, and healing gifts!

The Truth is in the Air

This blend of essential oils has been reported to open people up to having deep and honest conversations with one another. When you need to hear the truth about a certain situation from someone who loves you, this is the blend you will want to run in your diffuser.

Yield: 1 application

RECIPE

3 drops basil oil

2 drops pink grapefruit oil

2 drops ylang-ylang oil

Water

Follow your directions for using essential oils in your particular brand of diffuser. Ensure that your diffuser does not use heat but runs by vibration, sound waves, or another cold-steam type of process. Choose the essential oils needed for your condition, then add water and oils to the diffuser. Run your diffuser as needed to permeate the air with therapeutic properties and achieve the results you desire.

Truth Serum Roller

This makes an easy-to-carry essential oil blend that smells so good that people will think it is perfume. Keep the conversations and communications honest by applying this beforehand, and you can more easily tell and receive the truth with an open mind.

Yield: 1 fluid ounce

RECIPE

3 drops cassia oil

3 drops cypress oil

3 drops vetiver oil

3 drops vitamin E oil

1 fluid ounce carrier oil

Place the ingredients into a roller bottle. Roll around the area desired, such as wrist, neck, temples, soles of feet, or chest. You may also combine into a small bowl and apply to area with fingertips. Do not apply to open wounds, mucus membranes, eyes, or sensitive areas. Shake well before each use. Store unused portion in a glass jar or container with a tight-fitting lid in a cool, dark area for up to 3 months.

See Through Me Massage

With this massage and blend of essential oils, it is hard to deceive or be deceived. Concentrate on the one thing that you want a definitive answer to from yourself while receiving this massage. By the time you are done, you will be closer to knowing what you need to do.

Yield: 1 fluid ounce

RECIPE

6 drops frankincense oil

3 drops geranium oil

2 drops vetiver oil

2 drops ylang-ylang oil

2 drops basil oil

1 fluid ounce carrier oil

Pour the essential oils and the carrier oil into a small glass container, bowl, or jar. Swirl to mix the ingredients and use to massage lightly the area desired, such as temples, neck, chest, back, or soles of feet. Keep essential oil mixture away from open wounds, mucus membranes, genitals, eyes, and sensitive areas. Repeat application as needed. Store unused portion in a glass jar or container with a tight-fitting lid in a cool, dark area for up to 3 months.

The Truth is in the Bath

The essential oils in this bath will open the lines of communication to honest and forthright answers with either yourself or your partner.

Yield: 1 application

RECIPE

6 drops pink grapefruit oil

5 drops melissa oil

4 drops orange oil

2 tablespoons carrier oil

1 tablespoon milk (optional for adults, recommended for children)

As you begin to fill the tub with water, pour the chosen essential oils and carrier oil into the running water. Run a warm, not hot, bath. Water that is too hot will cause the essential oils to dissipate. You may add 1 tablespoon of milk to the water; this ensures that the essential oils will not stick to your skin, but will mix with the water. You may soak in the water as long as you are comfortable. Dry your feet well once you get out of the water, as the oils will cause them to be slippery, increasing your chances of falling. Rinse the tub of any remaining oils.

Luck

When fortune falls to us, we say, "That was good luck," but when bad things happen, we blame it on bad luck. There are essential oils derived from plants that have been believed to bring good luck to people for centuries. Try dabbing on a little and see how your luck changes.

Essential Oils
Frankincense, ginger, lime, patchouli, sandalwood, and spikenard

Good Luck Spray
Any time you feel like you need a little luck on your side, use this spray. These oils have been used in rituals and lotions for years, reportedly bringing good luck to the wearer.

Yield: 2 fluid ounces

RECIPE
4 drops frankincense oil
5 drops spikenard oil
6 drops patchouli oil
1 tablespoon witch hazel
2 fluid ounces water
3 drops vitamin E oil

Add all ingredients to a dark-colored spray bottle. Check for material steadfastness before spraying on fabric. Shake the bottle and spray onto area desired, such as body, hair, home, car, or office. Do not spray into or on open wounds, genitals, eyes, or mucus membranes. Store in a cool, dark area for up to 3 months. Shake well before each use to combine the ingredients.

Lucky Bath

When it feels like everything is going wrong, this is the bath to take that will turn your luck around. These essential oils have been used for many years to bring good luck into a person's life.

Yield: 1 application

RECIPE
3 drops lime oil
3 drops sandalwood oil
3 drops ginger oil
3 drops frankincense oil
1 tablespoon carrier oil
1 tablespoon milk (optional for adults, recommended for children)

As you begin to fill the tub with water, pour the chosen essential oils and carrier oil into the running water. Run a warm, not hot, bath. Water that is too hot will cause the essential oils to dissipate. You may add 1 tablespoon of milk to the water; this ensures that the essential oils will not stick to your skin, but will mix with the water. You may soak in the water as long as you are comfortable. Dry your feet well once you get out of the water, as the oils will cause them to be slippery, increasing your chances of falling. Rinse the tub of any remaining oils.

Lucky in Love Linen Powder

Combining both the essential oils for luck and the essential oils for love can only lead to good things. This linen powder has reputed lucky oils in it as well as calming, aphrodisiac, soothing, and relaxing oils. Wake up feeling like the tide has turned and luck is finally on your side.

Yield: ½ cup

RECIPE

7 drops frankincense oil

7 drops spikenard oil

7 drops sandalwood oil

½ cup cornstarch

4 drops vitamin E oil

Place the ingredients into a mason jar, stirring well with a whisk. Carefully poke holes into the lid, use this as a shaker, and shake the ingredients into pillowcases or under sheet areas as needed. You can get a piece of plastic wrap and place it over the jar and under the lid to keep powder from spilling out when not in use. Store in a glass jar or container with a tight-fitting lid in a cool, dark, and dry area for up to 3 months.

Lucky Chance Bath Salts

While soaking in this tub, you are supposed to concentrate on your luck turning around and getting what you want. Relax and let positive influences give you the visualization of your future exactly how you want it. These essential oils have been used for many years to increase your chances of bringing that visualized future to fruition and to also bring you the good luck you need to achieve it!

Yield: 3 cups

RECIPE

7 drops lime oil

7 drops ginger oil

7 drops spikenard oil

2 tablespoons carrier oil

5 drops vitamin E oil

3 cups salts

1 tablespoon milk (optional for adults, recommended for children)

Use any type of salt you prefer: pink Himalayan salt, sea salt, Epsom salts, etc. In a small container, add the essential oils to the desired type of salt. Stir until well blended. Screw lid onto container tightly. Leave mixture in a dark area for 24 hours and then stir mixture again. Run the bathwater. Once the tub is full of water, you can add the milk, and then add ½ cup of the bath salt mixture to bathwater as you get into the tub. You may stay in the tub as long as the temperature is comfortable. Dry your feet well when you get out of the bath, as the oils are slippery and can cause you to fall. Store remainder in a glass jar or container with a tight-fitting lid in a cool, dark area for up to 3 months. These jars make attractive, inexpensive, and healing gifts!

Patience

We all desire patience in ourselves and in others. Patience is a virtue that takes time to acquire, and most of us are not born with it. Essential oils can help a person control their emotions and not be so quick to anger. These essential oils have been used for a long time to quell the impulsive and oftentimes adverse emotions that want to take over. The calming, relaxing components of these oils reduce anxiety and anger and bring that calm "wait-it-out" feeling that we all need from time to time.

Essential Oils

Bergamot, geranium, lavender, neroli, patchouli, rose, and ylang-ylang

Patience Powder

This is the perfect recipe to bring you patience while you sleep. Sprinkle it under your sheets so that you can fall asleep quickly and wake up with loving, calm, and peaceful intentions. The calming properties in this recipe include antidepressant, nervine, and sedative elements.

Yield: ¼ cup

RECIPE
3 drops lavender oil
3 drops rose oil
3 drops vetiver oil
4 drops vitamin E oil
¼ cup cornstarch

Place the ingredients into a mason jar, stirring well with a whisk. Carefully poke holes into the lid, use this as a shaker, and shake the ingredients into pillowcases or under sheet areas as needed. You can get a piece of plastic wrap and place it over the jar and under the lid to keep powder from spilling out when not in use. Store in a glass jar or container with a tight-fitting lid in a cool, dark, and dry area for up to 3 months.

Exquisite Rest Bath

When you are feeling exasperated and out of sorts, the essential oil combination in this bath will have you happy and relaxed and able to deal with the situation at hand. With patience, we can mull over the issues that are at the forefront of our minds and deal with problems in a more rational manner. This blend contains sedative, antidepressant, analgesic, grounding, and tonic properties.

Yield: 1 application

RECIPE
5 drops vetiver oil
5 drops neroli oil
5 drops bergamot oil
1 tablespoon carrier oil
1 tablespoon milk (optional for adults, recommended for children)

As you begin to fill the tub with water, pour the chosen essential oils and carrier oil into the running water. Run a warm, not hot, bath. Water that is too hot will cause the essential oils to dissipate. You may add 1 tablespoon of milk to the water; this ensures that the essential oils will not stick to your skin, but will mix with the water. You may soak in the water as long as you are comfortable. Dry your feet well once you get out of the water, as the oils will cause them to be slippery, increasing your chances of falling. Rinse the tub of any remaining oils.

Stop and Smell Inhale

This is perfect for those necessary visits to that government agency or at the doctor's office—when you know you will be getting impatient. Just whip out this little vial, take a whiff, and you will soon be relaxed and feeling fine. These oils contain sedative and tranquilizing properties that make waiting it out a blissful experience!

Yield: 1 application

Recipe
1 drop lavender oil

or

1 drop rose oil

Choose your essential oil and apply to the palm of your hand, an oil inhaler, or a tissue. Bring the essential oils close to your nostrils and inhale the aroma deeply. You can cover one nostril at a time with your thumb and, if you prefer, alternate nostrils. This process sends the properties straight to your brain and the effects are immediate. You can complete this procedure 3–4 times daily.

Fragrant Spritzer

When the kids are screaming, the partner won't help you out, and the dinner is burning, this spritzer will instantly take you from a crazy "at the end of your rope" maniac to one of those "this too shall pass" humans. You can do it! The elements at work here include antidepressant, sedative, calming, and tonic properties.

Yield: 2 fluid ounces

Recipe
9 drops rosewood oil
6 drops neroli oil
6 drops vetiver oil
5 drops vitamin E oil
2 fluid ounces water

Spritzers are lighter than sprays, and easier to wear on the body or in your hair. Mix the essential oils, water, and witch hazel into a spray bottle. Shake well before each use. Lightly spray the area desired, such as body, hair, clothing (check first for color damage to clothing and furniture), rooms, car, or office. The lightly scented fragrance and the healing therapeutic properties will soon make this one of your favorite methods of using your oils. Store your spritzer in a cool, dark area for up to 3 months.

I Am Zen Massage

This massage oil blend is perfect to use when your partner is feeling frustrated and impatient with the day's events. This is a great one for a "type B" personality to use on a "type A" personality when wanting to instill patience and calmness in your partner or yourself. What a soothing, relaxing, and perfect way to end your day. This blend includes sedative, aphrodisiac, and antidepressant properties.

Yield: 1 fluid ounce

RECIPE

8 drops patchouli oil

4 drops bergamot oil

4 drops ylang-ylang oil

4 drops vitamin E oil

1 fluid ounce carrier oil

Pour the essential oils and the carrier oil into a small glass container, bowl, or jar. Swirl to mix the ingredients and use to massage lightly the area desired, such as temples, neck, chest, back, or soles of feet. Keep essential oil mixture away from open wounds, mucus membranes, genitals, eyes, and sensitive areas. Repeat application as needed. Store unused portion in a glass jar or container with a tight-fitting lid in a cool, dark area for up to 3 months.

Chill Out Diffuser

This diffuser recipe is wonderful to use to calm and relax even the most impatient person. Run it at work, in the office, or anywhere people gather to talk negatively. They will soon be offering compliments and smiling when the air is infused with this aroma that is infused with aphrodisiac, antidepressant, and calming therapeutic properties.

Yield: 1 application

RECIPE

4 drops neroli oil

3 drops rosewood oil

3 drops rose oil

2 drops geranium oil

Water

Follow your directions for using essential oils in your particular brand of diffuser. Ensure that your diffuser does not use heat but runs by vibration, sound waves, or another cold-steam type of process. Choose the essential oils needed for your condition, then add water and oils to the diffuser. Run your diffuser as needed to permeate the air with therapeutic properties and achieve the results you desire.

 Peace

Almost everyone desires peace in his or her life and for others in the world. Essential oils can bring about a sense of peace, calm, and relaxation in your life and in the lives of those you surround yourself with. Whether through bathing yourself with essential oils, or diffusing a room to bring peace to others, achieving this contented feeling is tantamount to a happy life.

Essential Oils

German chamomile, lavender, myrrh, myrtle, and neroli

Peace Powder

Sprinkle this essential oil recipe under everyone's sheets and you will have the entire family getting along and mending fences while, at the same time, you can acquire a peaceful night's sleep. These essential oils have sedative, antidepressant, and tranquilizing properties.

Yield: ¼ cup

RECIPE

3 drops German chamomile oil

3 drops lavender oil

3 drops myrtle oil

4 drops vitamin E oil

¼ cup cornstarch

Place the ingredients into a mason jar, stirring well with a whisk. Carefully poke holes into the lid, use this as a shaker, and shake the ingredients into pillowcases or under sheet areas as needed. You can get a piece of plastic wrap and place it over the jar and under the lid to keep powder from spilling out when not in use. Store in a glass jar or container with a tight-fitting lid in a cool, dark, and dry area for up to 3 months.

Blowing Wind Bath Salts

This is the perfect recipe to use after you have had an argument and the stress is eating you up. Give your brain and your overactive mind a rest. You will forget about everything as you relax and melt into this bath with its sedative, tranquilizing, and antidepressant properties.

Yield: 3 cups

RECIPE

7 drops neroli oil

7 drops German chamomile oil

7 drops myrtle oil

5 drops vitamin E oil

2 tablespoons carrier oil

3 cups salts

1 tablespoon milk (optional for adults, recommended for children)

Use any type of salt you prefer: pink Himalayan salt, sea salt, Epsom salts, etc. In a small container, add the essential oils to the desired type of salt. Stir until well blended. Screw lid onto container tightly. Leave mixture in a dark area for 24 hours and then stir mixture again. Run the bathwater. Once the tub is full of water, you can add the milk, and then add ½ cup of the bath salt mixture to bathwater as you get into the tub. You may stay in the tub as long as the temperature is comfortable. Dry your feet well when you get out of the bath, as the oils are slippery and can cause you

to fall. Store remainder in a glass jar or container with a tight-fitting lid in a cool, dark area for up to 3 months. These jars make attractive, inexpensive, and healing gifts!

Peaceful Spray

Fill the air in your home with positive energy and peace and instill patience in yourself with this essential oil spray. These oils contain cordial, sedative, antidepressant, and aphrodisiac therapeutic properties.

Yield: 2 fluid ounces

RECIPE
9 drops lavender oil
13 drops neroli oil
1 tablespoon witch hazel
2 fluid ounces water

Add all ingredients to a dark-colored spray bottle. Check for material steadfastness before spraying on fabric. Shake the bottle and spray onto area desired, such as body, hair, home, car, or office. Do not spray into or on open wounds, genitals, eyes, or mucus membranes. Store in a cool, dark area for up to 3 months. Shake well before each use to combine the ingredients.

Pranayama Air

Run this diffuser recipe to banish the negative energy and replace it with positive energy and peace. These oils contain sedative, relaxing, antispasmodic, and nervine properties.

Yield: 1 application

RECIPE
5 drops myrtle oil
5 drops German chamomile oil
Water

Follow your directions for using essential oils in your particular brand of diffuser. Ensure that your diffuser does not use heat but runs by vibration, sound waves, or an-

other cold-steam type of process. Choose the essential oils needed for your condition, then add water and oils to the diffuser. Run your diffuser as needed to permeate the air with therapeutic properties and achieve the results you desire.

Mindfulness Inhale

Keep a vial of one of these essential oils handy, and when outside forces cause you to feel stressed, take a smell of the oils in your vial and you will be enveloped with a sense of peace. The nervine, sedative, and antidepressant properties will relax and uplift your spirit.

Yield: 1 application

RECIPE
1 drop lavender oil

or

1 drop neroli oil

Choose your essential oil and apply to the palm of your hand, an oil inhaler, or a tissue. Bring the essential oils close to your nostrils and inhale the aroma deeply. You can cover one nostril at a time with your thumb and, if you prefer, alternate nostrils. This process sends the properties straight to your brain and the effects are immediate. You can complete this procedure 3–4 times daily.

All Is One Bath

When conflict, tension, and everyday stress have you at each other's throats, this is the bath that will bring you back together. Surround yourself with the soothing, peaceful aromas and agents in this blend. This recipe contains therapeutic properties such as aphrodisiac, sedative, and tonic components.

Yield: 1 application

RECIPE
5 drops lavender oil
5 drops neroli oil

5 drops myrtle oil

1 tablespoon carrier oil

1 tablespoon milk (optional for adults, recommended for children)

As you begin to fill the tub with water, pour the chosen essential oils and carrier oil into the running water. Run a warm, not hot, bath. Water that is too hot will cause the essential oils to dissipate. You may add 1 tablespoon of milk to the water; this ensures that the essential oils will not stick to your skin, but will mix with the water. You may soak in the water as long as you are comfortable. Dry your feet well once you get out of the water, as the oils will cause them to be slippery, increasing your chances of falling. Rinse the tub of any remaining oils.

Prosperity

To be prosperous means to have obtained a comfortable station in life and to be receiving all that one needs. This could pertain to wealth, health, status, spirituality, mentality, love, or in any number of ways a person may consider themselves to "have it all." Essential oils, herbs, plants, and flowers have been used for thousands of years to help a person to obtain and secure their prosperity.

Essential Oils

Almond, allspice, bergamot, cinnamon, clove, frankincense, helichrysum, myrrh, patchouli, orange, sandalwood, spikenard, spruce, and vetiver

Wear It Well Laundry Detergent

Take these essential oils with you everywhere you go by laundering your clothing in them. These oils are favorites by many people who have used them for generations for the intention of obtaining and securing prosperous lives.

Yield: ¼ cup

RECIPE

2 drops bergamot oil

2 drops sandalwood oil

¼ cup liquid laundry detergent

Mix the ingredients together in a small bowl or container. Stir well. Add the manufacturer's recommended amount of oil-infused detergent to each load in the washer. Store remainder in a glass jar with a tight-fitting lid in a cool, dark area for up to 1 year.

Journey Wrist Rub

This little gem of a recipe is what I have been using for years when I feel like everything is going south! These oils are reportedly used to help make one prosperous in all of the areas that they desire. This blend also smells really good, so I get compliments on my "perfume" when wearing this.

Yield: 1 fluid ounce

RECIPE

4 drops orange oil

3 drops bergamot oil

2 drops frankincense oil

2 drops ginger oil

3 drops vitamin E oil

1 fluid ounce carrier oil

Pour the essential oils, carrier oil, and any remaining ingredients into a small glass container, bowl, or jar. Swirl or whisk to mix the ingredients and apply lightly to the area desired, such as pressure points, wrists, neck, soles of feet, temples or chest. Keep essential oil mixture away from open wounds, mucus membranes, genitals, eyes, and sensitive areas. Repeat application as needed, usually 2–3 times daily. You may cover area with linen or cloth to protect clothing and furniture. Store unused portion in a glass jar or container with a tight-fitting lid in a cool, dark area for up to 3 months.

I Can Have It All Spritzer

There is no need to feel you can't have it all! Love, career, health, money, inner peace, and all sorts of prosperous means are yours for the asking. These essential oils are reported to bring us everything we desire. Spray this prosperity spritzer everywhere you wish to succeed … even on yourself.

Yield: 2 fluid ounces

R ECIPE
7 drops helichrysum oil

7 drops myrrh oil

3 drops patchouli oil

2 drops spikenard oil

1 tablespoon witch hazel

2 fluid ounces water

Spritzers are lighter than sprays, and easier to wear on the body or in your hair. Mix the essential oils, water, and witch hazel into a spray bottle. Shake well before each use. Lightly spray the area desired, such as body, hair, clothing (check first for color damage to clothing and furniture), rooms, car, or office. The lightly scented fragrance and the healing therapeutic properties will soon make this one of your favorite methods of using your oils. Store your spritzer in a cool, dark area for up to 3 months.

Prosperity Roll-On

This recipe contains the oils that have been believed to bring prosperity to the wearer. This recipe is easy to make, use, and carry so that you can have it at a moment's notice. It helps the wearer to feel a shield of protection. These essential oils bring a sense of calm and relief, dispelling anxiety and worry. This roller bottle is handy to carry in your car or purse so that when you are feeling the need, it can be put on in moments.

R ECIPE
3 drops helichrysum oil

3 drops orange oil

3 drops bergamot oil

2 drops vitamin E oil

1 fluid ounce carrier oil

Place the ingredients into a roller bottle. Roll around the area desired, such as wrist, neck, temples, soles of feet, or chest. Do not apply to open wounds, mucus membranes, eyes, or sensitive areas. Shake well before each use. Store unused portion in a glass jar or container with a tight-fitting lid in a cool, dark area for up to 3 months.

Romance

Using aromas to add an element of romance to our lives is so natural that we do it all the time without even thinking about it: adding scented lotions to our daily repertoire, using perfume, scented soaps, bubble baths, candles, the list is endless of what we will do to make ourselves more attractive to our partners, and to get them in the mood for romance. Essential oils help in that they not only have some of the most fragrant aromas on earth, but that they actually have natural chemical compounds in them that attract our mates through pheromones and therapeutic properties such as aphrodisiac, sedative, calming, and antianxiety agents. When attempting to woo someone else, essential oils are an aid you can't do without. These are some of the oldest recipes known to the human race … Now they are yours!

Essential Oils

Angelica, bergamot, clary sage, jasmine, lime, mandarin, neroli, parsley, patchouli, Roman chamomile, rose, sandalwood, and ylang-ylang

Love Me Linen Spray

This powerful linen spray has all the ingredients to ensure a romantic night with your significant other. Spray this when you know your partner may need a little romance-booster in their life. This spray has so many great-feeling, all-natural, healthy, non-chemical pheromones to give that certain someone a nudge in the right direction.

Yield: 2 fluid ounces

RECIPE
5 drops rose oil
5 drops neroli oil
5 drops Roman chamomile oil
1 fluid ounce distilled water
1 fluid ounce vodka

Add all ingredients to a dark-colored spray bottle. Check for material steadfastness before spraying on fabric. Shake the bottle and spray onto area desired, such as body, hair, home, car, or office. Do not spray into or on open wounds, genitals, eyes, or mucus membranes. Store in a cool, dark area for up to 1 year. Shake well before each use to combine the ingredients.

Exotic Embrace Aromas Spray

Your clothing will smell great and attract your potential romantic partner with ease when this recipe is added to your daily routine. These oils will adhere to your clothing and leave a lingering scent long after you leave. Try this recipe on yourself and get that attention you have been waiting for. You will be surprised at your uplifted mood as a bonus!

Yield: 2 fluid ounces

RECIPE
5 drops mandarin oil
5 drops bergamot oil
5 drops lime oil
1 fluid ounce distilled water
1 fluid ounce vodka

Add all ingredients to a dark-colored spray bottle. Check for material steadfastness before spraying on fabric. Shake the bottle and spray onto area desired, such as body, hair, home, car, or office. Do not spray into or on open wounds, genitals, eyes, or mucus membranes. Store in a cool, dark area for up to 3 months. Shake well before each use to combine the ingredients.

Come Hither Roll-On

Try making a little of this blend that has aphrodisiacal elements in the essential oils to bring whomever you desire straight to your arms. This roll-on can be carried in your purse for easy access or left in a desk drawer at work. The natural romance will reportedly blossom with just a little dab on your wrists or throat.

Yield: 1 fluid ounce

RECIPE
7 drops rose oil
3 drops clary sage oil

2 drops ylang-ylang oil

2 drops sandalwood oil

3 drops vitamin E oil

1 tablespoon carrier oil

Place the ingredients into a roller bottle. Roll around the area desired, such as wrist, neck, temples, soles of feet, or chest. Do not apply to open wounds, mucus membranes, eyes, or sensitive areas. Shake well before each use. Store unused portion in a glass jar or container with a tight-fitting lid in a cool, dark area for up to 3 months.

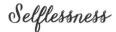 *Selflessness*

Selfless service is something that quite a few people have attempted, but few in this world can continue indefinitely with selfless acts. I, myself, have a constant battle within, attempting to continue acts of selfless service for others. Life and selfishness often get in the way. I like to use these recipes during times of prayer and meditation about how I can be of more service to others in this world. These oils have long been tied to various religions who are strident givers of themselves to others.

Essential Oils

Angelica, bay laurel, frankincense, jasmine, lemon, lotus, myrrh, orange, and rose

Gifts of Service Aroma

When I start to feel selfish and want to turn around by giving more of myself to others, whether it be my husband, my family and friends, or to those less fortunate, I use this diffuser recipe while praying or working, and it often helps me to give from myself to others.

Yield: 1 application

RECIPE

4 drops frankincense oil

4 drops myrrh oil

Water

Follow your directions for using essential oils in your particular brand of diffuser. Ensure that your diffuser does not use heat but runs by vibration, sound waves, or another cold-steam type of process. Choose the essential oils needed for your condition, then add water and oils to the diffuser. Run your diffuser as needed to permeate the air with therapeutic properties and achieve the results you desire.

Giver's Inhale

This inhalation of essential oils will open your heart and soul to giving of yourself to others. Selfless acts require nothing more than your care, your desire to help, and your time. When feeling stressed about what you are doing, just smell this aroma and let your heart take over. The best way to feel good about yourself is to make someone else feel happy about themselves.

Yield: 1 application

RECIPE
1 drop lotus oil

or

1 drop angelica oil

Choose your essential oil and apply to the palm of your hand, an oil inhaler, or a tissue. Bring the essential oils close to your nostrils and inhale the aroma deeply. You can cover one nostril at a time with your thumb and, if you prefer, alternate nostrils. This process sends the properties straight to your brain and the effects are immediate. You can complete this procedure 3–4 times daily.

Serenity

Serenity is often defined as a feeling of peace, calm, and bliss. Serenity can be obtained by many contributing factors such as meditation, family, nature, and happiness of career. Many people use these essential oils to help obtain the feeling of serenity and bliss due to the euphoric properties contained within these oils.

Essential Oils

Angelica, clary sage, eucalyptus, German chamomile, lavender, marjoram, peppermint, Roman chamomile, sandalwood, vanilla, and ylang-ylang

Serene Powder

When feeling frazzled and too frantic to sleep, apply a powder of these essential oils under the sheets to guarantee a serene night's sleep with its sedative, calming, and depurative properties.

Yield: ¼ cup

RECIPE
10 drops angelica oil
5 drops clary sage oil
¼ cup cornstarch

Place the ingredients into a mason jar, stirring well with a whisk. Carefully poke holes into the lid, use this as a shaker, and shake the ingredients into pillowcases or under sheet areas as needed. You can get a piece of plastic wrap and place it over the jar and under the lid to keep powder from spilling out when not in use. Store in a glass jar or container with a tight-fitting lid in a cool, dark, and dry area for up to 3 months.

Whispering Bath Salts

Not only will the salts have your body and your mind luxuriating in this bath, but the essential oils will help you to soothe your spirit and soul and bring back the grounding serenity you need. Angelica contains sedative and calming properties to relax you and bring peaceful, positive energy your way.

Yield: 3 cups

RECIPE
10 drops angelica oil
8 drops Roman chamomile oil
2 tablespoons carrier oil

3 cups salts

1 tablespoon milk (optional for adults, recommended for children)

Use any type of salt you prefer: pink Himalayan salt, sea salt, Epsom salts, etc. In a small container, add the essential oils to the desired type of salt. Stir until well blended. Screw lid onto container tightly. Leave mixture in a dark area for 24 hours and then stir mixture again. Run the bathwater. Once the tub is full of water, you can add the milk, and then add ½ cup of the bath salt mixture to bathwater as you get into the tub. You may stay in the tub as long as the temperature is comfortable. Dry your feet well when you get out of the bath, as the oils are slippery and can cause you to fall. Store remainder in a glass jar or container with a tight-fitting lid in a cool, dark area for up to 3 months. These jars make attractive, inexpensive, and healing gifts!

Om Spray

Carry this spray to work with you, and when everything around you is falling apart, compose yourself and remain above all the fray and serene with a healthy spray of this essential oil. These oils' calming and sedative properties will relax not only you but those who come into contact with you as well.

Yield: 2 fluid ounces

RECIPE

5 drops angelica oil

5 drops sandalwood oil

5 drops peppermint oil

1 tablespoon witch hazel

2 fluid ounces water

Add all ingredients to a dark-colored spray bottle. Check for material steadfastness before spraying on fabric. Shake the bottle and spray onto area desired, such as body, hair, home, car, or office. Do not spray into or on open wounds, genitals, eyes, or mucus membranes. Store in a cool, dark area for up to 3 months. Shake well before each use to combine the ingredients.

Serenity River Inhale

When you just desperately need a moment of serenity and clarity, this aroma will do the trick with its calming and sedative therapeutic properties.

Yield: 1 application

RECIPE

1 drop angelica oil

or

1 drop myrrh oil

Choose your essential oil and apply to the palm of your hand, an oil inhaler, or a tissue. Bring the essential oils close to your nostrils and inhale the aroma deeply. You can cover one nostril at a time with your thumb and, if you prefer, alternate nostrils. This process sends the properties straight to your brain and the effects are immediate. You can complete this procedure 3–4 times daily.

Vitality

We all wish for vitality in our lives: passion, strength, vigor, and an active spirit. There are multiple tasks each day that we can do to achieve vitality, such as eating well, exercise, communicating our needs, friendships, natural healing, and herbs. Essential oils have long been thought to bring vigor and fire back into a person's life. Vitality can be lost through illness, aging, divorce, boredom, death of a loved one, or any one of a thousand reasons. Try some of these recipes to help you restore that capacity to live life to the fullest and resurrect your youthful vitality.

Essential Oils

Bay laurel, bergamot, cinnamon leaf, eucalyptus, geranium, German chamomile, lemon, myrtle, orange, patchouli, peppermint, pink grapefruit, rose, sage, spearmint, tangerine, wintergreen, and ylang-ylang

Vitality Bath and Shower Bombs

This recipe brings laughter, youthfulness, and strong, active emotions to the user. Bath bombs are so popular because they bring exuberance to an otherwise mundane experience. Couple that with life-enhancing essential oils and you will have a treat to remember.

Yield: 8–12 bombs

RECIPE

1 cup baking soda

½ cup citric acid

½ cup cornstarch

½ cup Epsom salts, fine grained

8 drops orange oil

8 drops pink grapefruit oil

8 drops rose oil

½ teaspoon carrier oil

¾ teaspoon water

spray bottle (water)

In a large bowl, mix your dry ingredients together until fine with a whisk. In a tiny jar with a lid, add your wet ingredients and shake to mix. You may add a couple drops of food coloring to the wet jar. Extremely slowly, add the wet ingredients to the dry ingredients while whisking rapidly. If fizzing takes place, whisk until it is mixed. Once the ingredients are well mixed, it should be the texture of slightly damp sand. Add a spray or two of water if needed. Once the mixture is the consistency you like, form into balls; I just smash mine down into ice cube trays or muffin tins. You can use cute molds, but you must work rapidly as mixture will dry out quickly. Leave in open air, uncovered, in a room where they will not be disturbed for 12–24 hours. Once they are dry, you can place 1–2 bombs into your bath or directly into the spray of the shower and they will fizz and release their aromatic and healing properties. Store unused portion in an airtight container for up to 6 months.

Vitality Lip Balm

When wearing this lip balm, you will feel strong, active, and energetic. Increase your vitality by using essential oils that have the vigorous properties to help you feel more alive, energetic, and spontaneous.

Yield: 1 tablespoon

RECIPE

3 teaspoons grape seed oil

½ teaspoon beeswax pellets

4 drops vitamin E oil

3 drops spearmint oil

3 drops pink grapefruit oil

Heat the grape seed oil and the wax in a very small glass container in the microwave for 1½ minutes. Open the door every 15 seconds to avoid popping and splattering. Melt the beeswax and the carrier oil in a glass bowl in the microwave until most of the beeswax is melted. You can also use a pan on the stovetop on low. Cool slightly. Add the vitamin E and the essential oils and stir or whisk quickly. With a spoon, drip a drop of the mixture onto the counter and Let set for 1 minute. Pull your finger through the drop and check for consistency. If mixture is too thin, add more beeswax; if it is too thick, add more oil. Once desired consistency is acquired, immediately pour into small balm container (glass or metal) with a lid. After mixture cools, cover and store in a cool, dark area for up to 6 months.

I Am Fire Spritzer

This spritzer recipe will have you feeling strong and sure of yourself. The essential oils in this blend contain energizing properties to promote vitality and life.

Yield: 1 fluid ounce

RECIPE

6 drops tangerine oil

5 drops ylang-ylang oil

4 drops cinnamon leaf oil

1 teaspoon witch hazel

1 fluid ounce water

Spritzers are lighter than sprays, and easier to wear on the body or in your hair. Mix the essential oils, water, and witch hazel into a spray bottle. Shake well before each use. Lightly spray the area desired, such as body, hair, clothing (check first for color damage to clothing and furniture), rooms, car, or office. The lightly scented fragrance and the healing therapeutic properties will soon make this one of your favorite methods of using your oils. Store your spritzer in a cool, dark area for up to 3 months.

Wealth

We all want it, but few of us have it. For many years people have been said to have used the following recipes to acquire wealth. Maybe your power of belief plays a big part in the usage of essential oils to obtain wealth, but why not give it a shot? Professing gratitude for wealth while using this recipe would be the optimal way to approach the acquisition of wealth.

Essential Oils

Basil, bergamot, cinnamon, clove, dill, ginger, jasmine, neroli, patchouli, pine, and vetiver

Money, Money Bath Salts

This is an ages-old recipe that uses essential oils that are known for their abilities to help you attain the wealth you need to survive and thrive. You must also believe it will happen and thank your higher power every day you soak in this therapeutic bath.

Yield: 3 cups

RECIPE

7 drops ginger oil

7 drops dill oil

7 drops pine oil

2 tablespoons carrier oil

3 cups salts

1 tablespoon milk (optional for adults, recommended for children)

Use any type of salt you prefer: pink Himalayan salt, sea salt, Epsom salts, etc. In a small container, add the essential oils to the desired type of salt. Stir until well blended. Screw lid onto container tightly. Leave mixture in a dark area for 24 hours and then stir mixture again. Run the bathwater. Once the tub is full of water, you can add the milk, and then add ½ cup of the bath salt mixture to bathwater as you get into the tub. You may stay in the tub as long as the temperature is comfortable. Dry your feet well when you get out of the bath, as the oils are slippery and can cause you to fall. Store remainder in a glass jar or container with a tight-fitting lid in a cool, dark area for up to 3 months. These jars make attractive, inexpensive, and healing gifts!

Wealthy Powder

Sleep on this powder and perhaps you will wake up with *the* idea that will change the world and make you a billionaire. These essential oils have been used many times for people who want to make it big in life. Be sure that you say your thanks of gratitude while sleeping on this blend of money-making oils.

Yield: ¼ cup

RECIPE

3 drops pine oil

3 drops bergamot oil

3 drops neroli oil

4 drops vitamin E oil

¼ cup cornstarch

Place the ingredients into a mason jar, stirring well with a whisk. Carefully poke holes into the lid, use this as a shaker, and shake the ingredients into pillowcases or under sheet areas as needed. You can get a piece of plastic wrap and place it over the jar and under the lid to keep powder from spilling out when not in use. Store in a glass jar or container with a tight-fitting lid in a cool, dark, and dry area for up to 3 months.

A Wealthy Air

Run this diffuser recipe to fill your home with essential oils reported to bring wealth to families. When you breathe in this aroma, remember to be respectful and thankful to Spirit for your successes and failures.

Yield: 1 application

RECIPE
3 drops basil oil
3 drops vetiver oil
3 drops bergamot oil
Water

Follow your directions for using essential oils in your particular brand of diffuser. Ensure that your diffuser does not use heat but runs by vibration, sound waves, or another cold-steam type of process. Choose the essential oils needed for your condition, then add water and oils to the diffuser. Run your diffuser as needed to permeate the air with therapeutic properties and achieve the results you desire.

Inhale the $

Are you about to go to a great job interview? Play at the casino? Buy a lottery ticket? Smelling basil oil has been thought for thousands of years to bring about money luck. Be grateful, thankful, and appreciative of all that you have … and all that you will receive.

Yield: 1 application

RECIPE
1 drop basil oil

Choose your essential oil and apply to the palm of your hand, an oil inhaler, or a tissue. Bring the essential oils close to your nostrils and inhale the aroma deeply. You can cover one nostril at a time with your thumb and, if you prefer, alternate nostrils. This process sends the properties straight to your brain and the effects are immediate. You can complete this procedure 3–4 times daily.

Prosperity Bath

Bathe yourself in a bath that contains the essential oils that have been reported to draw wealth and success to many people. As you soak in this tub of success-accruing essential oils, whisper prayers of thanks and gratitude for that which you are about to receive.

Yield: 1 application

RECIPE

3 drops bergamot oil

3 drops vetiver oil

3 drops nutmeg oil

3 drops ginger oil

1 tablespoon carrier oil

1 tablespoon milk (optional for adults, recommended for children)

As you begin to fill the tub with water, pour the chosen essential oils and carrier oil into the running water. Run a warm, not hot, bath. Water that is too hot will cause the essential oils to dissipate. You may add 1 tablespoon of milk to the water; this ensures that the essential oils will not stick to your skin, but will mix with the water. You may soak in the water as long as you are comfortable. Dry your feet well once you get out of the water, as the oils will cause them to be slippery, increasing your chances of falling. Rinse the tub of any remaining oils.

Luxury Massage

If you're going to get a massage, why not luxuriate in one that uses essential oils reported to bring you financial stability? While receiving your massage, think about the blessings in your life, be grateful, and envision that which will soon come your way.

Yield: 1 fluid ounce

RECIPE

2 drops cinnamon oil

3 drops jasmine oil

2 drops patchouli oil

3 drops bergamot oil

3 drops vitamin E oil

1 fluid ounce carrier oil

Pour the essential oils and the carrier oil into a small glass container, bowl, or jar. Swirl to mix the ingredients and use to massage lightly the area desired, such as temples, neck, chest, back, or soles of feet. Keep essential oil mixture away from open wounds, mucus membranes, genitals, eyes, and sensitive areas. Repeat application as needed. Store unused portion in a glass jar or container with a tight-fitting lid in a cool, dark area for up to 3 months.

$pray $pray

Spray this everywhere and give yourself the chance to accumulate the wealth you have always dreamed of. Show your gratitude to your higher power each time you use this delightful blend; conceive, believe, and you shall receive.

Yield: 2 fluid ounces

RECIPE

10 drops neroli oil

2 drops dill oil

2 drops pine oil

4 drops jasmine oil

1 tablespoon witch hazel

2 fluid ounces water

Add all ingredients to a dark-colored spray bottle. Check for material steadfastness before spraying on fabric. Shake the bottle and spray onto area desired, such as body, hair, home, car, or office. Do not spray into or on open wounds, genitals, eyes, or mucus membranes. Store in a cool, dark area for up to 3 months. Shake well before each use to combine the ingredients.

Weight Reduction

Diet, heredity, health, and exercise play a huge part in someone keeping their weight under control. Essential oils can also play an important part by assisting someone in coping with their emotions and deterring an unhealthy diet choice. These recipes are also about helping a person increase their energy levels so that they will get up and move and burn off those unwanted calories. Essential oils can help in a variety of ways in the war against weight.

Essential Oils

Cinnamon, fennel, ginger, grapefruit, lemon, patchouli, and peppermint

Weight Loss Rub

These essential oils are derived from the plants most associated with weight loss. A few of the benefits in this recipe include antidepressant, aperitif, diuretic, and stimulant properties.

Yield: 1 fluid ounce

RECIPE
3 drops grapefruit oil
3 drops ginger oil
2 drops peppermint oil
1 drop lemon oil
5 drops vitamin E oil
1 fluid ounce carrier oil

Pour the essential oils, carrier oil, and any remaining ingredients into a small glass container, bowl, or jar. Swirl or whisk to mix the ingredients and apply lightly to the area desired, such as pressure points, neck, soles of feet, temples, or chest. Keep essential oil mixture away from open wounds, mucus membranes, genitals, eyes, and sensitive areas. Repeat application as needed, usually 2–3 times daily. You may cover area with linen or cloth to protect clothing and furniture. Store unused portion in a glass jar or container with a tight-fitting lid in a cool, dark area for up to 3 months.

Winning

Whether winning an event, a prize, or life, essential oils have been used to promote being a winner across the world. These are a couple of the essential oils that have been reputed to assist a person in winning and achieving that much sought-after goal.

Essential Oils

Bergamot, eucalyptus, lemon, lemongrass, neroli, orange, and spearmint

Winning Powder

I feel like every time I sleep on this particular powder blend, the next day a winning moment happens in my life. I am sharing this with you because I want you to experience those winning and fulfilling lifetime achievements as well.

Yield: ¼ cup

RECIPE
7 drops lemongrass oil
8 drops spearmint oil
4 drops vitamin E oil
¼ cup cornstarch

Place the ingredients into a mason jar, stirring well with a whisk. Carefully poke holes into the lid, use this as a shaker, and shake the ingredients into pillowcases or under sheet areas as needed. You can get a piece of plastic wrap and place it over the jar and under the lid to keep powder from spilling out when not in use. Store in a glass jar or container with a tight-fitting lid in a cool, dark, and dry area for up to 3 months.

Watch Me Now Bath Salts

Use this recipe in your bath when you're about to meet a new client or attend some event that you need an extra edge in. These essential oils have been derived from plants and used for centuries for their uplifting, energizing, and self-esteem–boosting properties.

Yield: 3 cups

RECIPE
9 drops neroli oil
9 drops bergamot oil
2 tablespoons carrier oil
3 cups salts
1 tablespoon milk (optional for adults, recommended for children)

Use any type of salt you prefer: pink Himalayan salt, sea salt, Epsom salts, etc. In a small container, add the essential oils to the desired type of salt. Stir until well blended. Screw lid onto container tightly. Leave mixture in a dark area for 24 hours and then stir mixture again. Run the bathwater. Once the tub is full of water, you can add the milk, and then add ½ cup of the bath salt mixture to bathwater as you get into the tub. You may stay in the tub as long as the temperature is comfortable. Dry your feet well when you get out of the bath, as the oils are slippery and can cause you to fall. Store remainder in a glass jar or container with a tight-fitting lid in a cool, dark area for up to 3 months. These jars make attractive, inexpensive, and healing gifts!

You Always Win

These essential oils have been reported to give an edge to someone who either inhales the aromas of the oils or applies them just before an event.

Yield: 1 application

RECIPE
1 drop lemon oil
or
1 drop eucalyptus oil

Choose your essential oil and apply to the palm of your hand, an oil inhaler, or a tissue. Bring the essential oils close to your nostrils and inhale the aroma deeply. You can cover one nostril at a time with your thumb and, if you prefer, alternate nostrils. This process sends the properties straight to your brain and the effects are immediate. You can complete this procedure 3–4 times daily.

I Won! Spray

You will be shouting "I won!" if you use this spray before you compete at a game, at an event, or at life.

Yield: 2 fluid ounces

RECIPE
6 drops bergamot oil
6 drops spearmint oil
6 drops patchouli oil
1 teaspoon vitamin E oil
1 tablespoon witch hazel
2 fluid ounces water

Add all ingredients to a dark-colored spray bottle. Check for material steadfastness before spraying on fabric. Shake the bottle and spray onto area desired, such as body, hair, home, car, or office. Do not spray into or on open wounds, genitals, eyes, or mucus membranes. Store in a cool, dark area for up to 3 months. Shake well before each use to combine the ingredients.

Wisdom

Clearing the mind of useless junk and filling the mind, soul, and spirit with wisdom has long been a goal of multitudes of people in every country and culture on earth throughout history. These essential oils have been reputed to help a person achieve the wisdom to fulfill their destinies.

Essential Oils

Cardamom, clary sage, cypress, sage, and vetiver

Wisdom Powder

This recipe uses essential oils that have been used for years and years to bring wisdom to those who inhale it. Use this blend when you wish to retain knowledge due to the memory-enhancing benefits of these oils. These oils work together to bring increasing wisdom to whomever sleeps on them.

Yield: ¼ cup

RECIPE
7 drops clary sage oil
3 drops cardamom oil
3 drops vetiver oil
4 drops vitamin E oil
¼ cup cornstarch

Place the ingredients into a mason jar, stirring well with a whisk. Carefully poke holes into the lid, use this as a shaker, and shake the ingredients into pillowcases or under sheet areas as needed. You can get a piece of plastic wrap and place it over the jar and under the lid to keep powder from spilling out when not in use. Store in a glass jar or container with a tight-fitting lid in a cool, dark, and dry area for up to 3 months.

Wise Old Owl Bath Salts

If you have a serious problem to ponder, take a bath with these essential oils and you could come out of your bath with a clear head and knowing the best route to take with your life and your decisions. Begin the process of being the solution.

Yield: 3 cups

RECIPE
7 drops vetiver oil
7 drops cardamom oil
7 drops clary sage oil
5 drops vitamin E oil
2 tablespoons carrier oil
3 cups salts
1 tablespoon milk (optional for adults, recommended for children)

Use any type of salt you prefer: pink Himalayan salt, sea salt, Epsom salts, etc. In a small container, add the essential oils to the desired type of salt. Stir until well blended. Screw lid onto container tightly. Leave mixture in a dark area for 24 hours and then stir mixture again. Run the bathwater. Once the tub is full of water, you can add the milk, and then add ½ cup of the bath salt mixture to bathwater as you get into the tub. You may stay in the tub as long as the temperature is comfortable. Dry your feet well when you get out of the bath, as the oils are slippery and can cause you to fall. Store remainder in a glass jar or container with a tight-fitting lid in a cool, dark area for up to 3 months. These jars make attractive, inexpensive, and healing gifts!

Wise Sage Inhale

Sometimes in our hectic daily schedules, we feel confused, foggy, and not able to think clearly. Maybe we aren't dedicating our lives to the pursuit of wisdom like the sages of the past, but it would be nice to be able to appear a little knowledgeable at times. This aroma will assist you with clarity of your mind and thoughts.

Yield: 1 application

RECIPE
1 drop clary sage oil

Choose your essential oil and apply to the palm of your hand, an oil inhaler, or a tissue. Bring the essential oils close to your nostrils and inhale the aroma deeply. You can cover one nostril at a time with your thumb and, if you prefer, alternate nostrils. This process sends the properties straight to your brain and the effects are immediate. You can complete this procedure 3–4 times daily.

Ancient Knowledge Spray

This spray reportedly works wonders for increasing your brain activity and enhancing your memory and your communication skills. This blend also has very pleasing aromatic attributes.

Yield: 2 fluid ounces

RECIPE
4 drops clary sage oil
4 drops vetiver oil

3 drops cardamom oil

1 tablespoon witch hazel

2 fluid ounces water

Add all ingredients to a dark-colored spray bottle. Check for material steadfastness before spraying on fabric. Shake the bottle and spray onto area desired, such as body, hair, home, car, or office. Do not spray into or on open wounds, genitals, eyes, or mucus membranes. Store in a cool, dark area for up to 3 months. Shake well before each use to combine the ingredients.

Brain Rebooting Bath

Take this bath once a month or more often to assist in keeping those brain cells working properly. These essential oils are extracted from plants that have been used for thousands of years in rituals known to increase wisdom and expand the mind.

Yield: 1 application

RECIPE

4 drops clary sage oil

3 drops cypress oil

3 drops cardamom oil

4 drops vetiver oil

1 tablespoon carrier oil

1 tablespoon milk (optional for adults, recommended for children)

As you begin to fill the tub with water, pour the chosen essential oils and carrier oil into the running water. Run a warm, not hot, bath. Water that is too hot will cause the essential oils to dissipate. You may add 1 tablespoon of milk to the water; this ensures that the essential oils will not stick to your skin, but will mix with the water. You may soak in the water as long as you are comfortable. Dry your feet well once you get out of the water, as the oils will cause them to be slippery, increasing your chances of falling. Rinse the tub of any remaining oils.

CHAPTER 7
Recipes for Devotion

*D*evotion comes in many shapes, forms, and areas of belief. Whether it is organized religion, personal convictions, or spiritual awakening, increasing your devotion is a practice long held by cultures across the span of time and distance. These oil and herbal recipes have been used since the dawn of man to increase one's ability to effectively increase devotion.

Beliefs

When doubt and fear plague our thoughts, sometimes our belief in something is shaken. To empower your beliefs and help you take a stand in what you believe in, apply some of these oils and blends that have been used for centuries to deepen and instill belief in ourselves, our passions, and our higher power.

Essential Oils

Angelica, bergamot, balsam fir, bay laurel, coriander, frankincense, geranium, jasmine, orange, rosemary, rosewood, and ylang-ylang

Wholehearted Spray

This spray is one that is used to reconnect with the universe, our higher power, and our beliefs. The components of sedative, antidepressant, nervine, and tonic properties work together to calm and provide peace.

Yield: 2 fluid ounces

RECIPE

9 drops bay laurel oil

5 drops ylang-ylang oil

5 drops balsam fir oil

2 fluid ounces water

1 tablespoon witch hazel

Add all ingredients to a dark-colored spray bottle. Check for material steadfastness before spraying on fabric. Shake the bottle and spray onto area desired. Do not spray into or on open wounds, genitals, eyes, or mucus membranes. Store in a cool, dark area for up to 3 months. Shake well before each use to combine the ingredients.

Empowerment Salve

This balm is good for my soul, spirit, and positivity as I go about my day. These essential oils are used for enhancing the spiritual experience and bringing back lost faith. Before I spend a day alone, cleaning, or completing chores, I like to use this balm and my thoughts turn repeatedly to faith, beliefs, meditation, and prayer. The sedative properties in this blend have a calming and relaxing effect on our mind and soul, while the tonic agents assist us in completing the tasks at hand.

Yield: 1 fluid ounce

RECIPE

1 fluid ounce carrier oil

1–2 ounces beeswax pellets

4 drops vitamin E oil

10 drops frankincense oil

10 drops angelica oil

Heat the beeswax and the carrier oil in a glass bowl in the microwave for 1½–2 minutes, until just melted, or on low on the stovetop. If you open the door every 15 seconds, you can avoid the popping of the wax and oil and overheating. Carefully remove the container from the microwave and stir. Drip a drop of the melted oil and wax onto the counter, after 1 minute check for consistency. If it is too thin, add more beeswax to the container; if it is too thick, add more carrier oil. Add the vitamin E oil and the essential oil to the heated mixture in the container. Whisk lightly, and it will begin hardening immediately. Pour into containers. Ensure your containers are glass or tin to prevent leeching of chemicals. Once cool, apply to wrists, temples, neck, or soles of feet. Do not apply to mucus membranes, eyes, genitals, or open wounds. Label containers and store in a dark, dry area for up to 1 year.

Renewing Beliefs Shower Bombs

Using these bath and shower bombs with these essential oils will have you feeling so positive, grateful, and thankful. This whole bath or shower experience is an awesome way to spend time alone with yourself and your higher power and bring your beliefs to the forefront of your thoughts. The antidepressant, aphrodisiac, and stimulating properties work together to uplift your spirit and well-being.

Yield: 12–18 bombs

RECIPE
1 cup baking soda
½ cup citric acid
½ cup cornstarch
½ cup Epsom salts, fine grained
15 drops coriander oil
15 drops bergamot oil
10 drops rosewood oil
½ teaspoon carrier oil
¾ teaspoon water
spray bottle (water)

In a large bowl, mix your dry ingredients together until fine with a whisk. In a tiny jar with a lid, add your wet ingredients and shake to mix. You may add a couple drops of food coloring to the wet jar. Extremely slowly, add the wet ingredients to the dry ingredients while whisking rapidly. If fizzing takes place, whisk until it is mixed. Once the ingredients are well mixed, it should be the texture of slightly damp sand. Add a spray or two of water if needed. Once the mixture is the consistency you like, form into balls; I just smash mine down into ice cube trays or muffin tins. You can use cute molds, but you must work rapidly as mixture will dry out quickly. Leave in open air, uncovered, in a room where they will not be disturbed for 12–24 hours. Once they are dry, you can place 1–2 bombs into your bath or directly into the spray of the shower and they will fizz and release their aromatic and healing properties. Store unused portion in an airtight container for up to 6 months.

Blessings

Whether asking for blessings for your family, yourself, your health, your life, or your home, blessings are nothing but good all around. These essential oils have been used all over the world in countless cultures, rituals, and religions to help with receiving and asking for blessings. I love to bless my home, my friend's homes, and hotel rooms and to ask for blessings for my family and my life. Give these recipes a try for yourself and your loved ones.

Essential Oils

Bergamot, cinnamon, frankincense, helichrysum, jasmine, juniper berry, lavender, mugwort, myrrh, patchouli, rose, rosemary, sandalwood, and spikenard

Home Blessing Anointing Oil

I like to use these oils if I feel negativity in my home. These oils are known for their cleansing and purifying properties. If someone is coming to visit, I usually spray this so that they will have a feeling of peace, contentment, and positivity, and they often comment on how zen my home feels! Therapeutic properties in these oils contain antidepressant, aphrodisiac, sedative, stimulating, and revitalizing natural agents. I often pray while mixing up this blend and ask Spirit to bless the oil.

Yield: 1 fluid ounce

RECIPE
5 drops patchouli oil
5 drops myrrh oil
5 drops jasmine oil
1 fluid ounce carrier oil

I like to use a thicker oil, such as olive oil, for this blend. Combine the ingredients in a dark-colored jar, preferably one with an eyedropper. Shake each time before use. I always pray and ask for only blessings and positivity while applying 1 drop of this blend to areas in the home, such as door frames, window sills, or headboards. Store remainder in a glass container, in a cool, dark area for up to 1 year.

Blessings Body Spray

This blend smells so lovely that not only will I receive blessings while wearing it, I will also smell a little like what I would imagine heaven smells like. The properties of this blend are spiritually uplifting with their antidepressant, aphrodisiac, sedative, tranquilizing, and relaxing components.

Yield: 2 fluid ounces

RECIPE
4 drops frankincense oil
4 drops vetiver oil
5 drops rose oil
3 drops mugwort oil
2 fluid ounces water
1 tablespoon witch hazel
3 drops vitamin E oil

Add all ingredients to a dark-colored spray bottle. Check for material steadfastness before spraying on fabric. Shake the bottle and spray onto area desired, I like to spray this on my yoga mat, in my bedroom, and anywhere where I want silence and peace. Do not spray into or on open wounds, genitals, eyes, or mucus membranes. Store in a cool, dark area for up to 3 months. Shake well before each use to combine the ingredients.

Personal Blessing Ointment

This blend is very special to me. I love to put a drop of this on my forehead before meditating or apply a drop to the soles of my feet. The properties in this blend are spiritual in nature, with their tonic and antidepressant components, and help me to keep focused and grounded while concentrating on blessings that I wish my loved ones, or myself, to receive. This blend is so wonderful that I often give it to those in need of a little prayer as a gift so that they can feel more open to asking for blessings for themselves.

Yield: 1 tablespoon

RECIPE
2 drops frankincense oil
2 drops helichrysum oil
2 drops sandalwood oil
2 drops vitamin E oil
1 tablespoon carrier oil

Combine ingredients into a small glass bowl, vial, or container with a lid. Apply 1 drop to pressure points on body such as soles of feet, neck, wrists, or temples. Store remainder in a cool, dark area for up to 3 months.

Blessings in the Air Diffuser

This diffuser blend has so many spiritual essential oils in it that your home or office will be filled with positivity and enlightenment. These essential oils are all spiritual in nature and will help you to receive the blessings you ask for.

Yield: 1 application

RECIPE
2 drops cypress oil
2 drops frankincense oil

2 drops spikenard oil

2 drops cedarwood oil

Water

Follow your directions for using essential oils in your particular brand of diffuser. Ensure that your diffuser does not use heat but runs by vibration, sound waves, or another cold-steam type of process. Choose the essential oils needed for your condition, then add water and oils to the diffuser. Run your diffuser as needed to permeate the air with therapeutic properties and achieve the results you desire.

Devotion

Devotion is a simple giving of one's self, mind, body, and soul to another person, belief, or project. Devotion requires a certain amount of passion for a particular belief. For example, many people are devoted to their children and will do anything in their power to ensure the child's safety, health, and success. Oftentimes our lack of devotion can lead to lethargy and apathy. Increasing one's devotion can be achieved with prayer, meditation, positive thoughts, and healing essential oils.

Essential Oils

Angelica, clary sage, frankincense, melissa, rose, sandalwood, and wild orange

Devotional Bath and Shower Bombs

These bath and shower bombs help to increase focus, positivity, and energy. Use one of them the next time you want to have complete devotion in a particular area. While relaxing in the bath, visualize the increase of your devotion and the outcome. I have made these bombs at the beginning of writing a particular book. I used them, soaked in the tub with them, prayed while in the tub, meditated on hopes and dreams while in the tub, and then made it happen with the devotion that developed in my spirit and soul.

Yield: 12–18 bombs

RECIPE

1 cup baking soda

½ cup citric acid

½ cup cornstarch
½ cup Epsom salts, fine grained
15 drops wild orange oil
15 drops sandalwood oil
½ teaspoon carrier oil
¾ teaspoon water
spray bottle (water)

In a large bowl, mix your dry ingredients together until fine with a whisk. In a tiny jar with a lid, add your wet ingredients and shake to mix. You may add a couple drops of food coloring to the wet jar. Extremely slowly, add the wet ingredients to the dry ingredients while whisking rapidly. If fizzing takes place, whisk until it is mixed. Once the ingredients are well mixed, it should be the texture of slightly damp sand. Add a spray or two of water if needed. Once the mixture is the consistency you like, form into balls; I just smash mine down into ice cube trays or muffin tins. You can use cute molds, but you must work rapidly as mixture will dry out quickly. Leave in open air, uncovered, in a room where they will not be disturbed for 12–24 hours. Once they are dry, you can place 1–2 bombs into your bath or directly into the spray of the shower and they will fizz and release their aromatic and healing properties. Store unused portion in an airtight container for up to 6 months.

Anointing Devotion

This simple recipe uses essential oils to help you to achieve that devotional spirit that focuses on embracing faith and matters of the soul. Working on our devotion to spiritual matters is of paramount importance in people's lives. Your soul and spirit are the basis for all that you are. These essential oils help to increase the ability to have the devotion needed to reach the next step in your journey, and to reach the next level of spirituality for your soul.

Yield: ½ ounce

RECIPE
5 drops melissa oil
5 drops angelica oil

3 drops vitamin E oil
½ ounce carrier oil

I like to use a thicker oil, such as olive oil, for this blend. Combine the ingredients in a dark-colored jar, preferably one with an eyedropper. Shake each time before use. I like to apply a drop of this to forehead, temples, neck, or soles of feet when meditating, doing yoga, praying, or for general good blessings. I always pray and ask for only blessings and positivity while applying one drop of this blend to areas in the home, such as door frames, windowsills, or headboards. Store remainder in a glass container, in a cool, dark area for up to 1 year.

Devoted Diffuser

Sometimes we may get the impression that our loved ones are not as devoted to us as we are to them. This diffuser can bring harmony to a household and have everyone caring for each other in devotion and peace. Use this recipe in times of discord and disconnect. These aromas and soothing therapeutic properties will bring about that connection that you have been longing for.

Yield: 1 application

RECIPE
5 drops rose oil
5 drops clary sage oil
Water

Follow your directions for using essential oils in your particular brand of diffuser. Ensure that your diffuser does not use heat but runs by vibration, sound waves, or another cold-steam type of process. Choose the essential oils needed for your condition, then add water and oils to the diffuser. Run your diffuser as needed to permeate the air with therapeutic properties and achieve the results you desire.

Faith

Faith is the ability to believe wholeheartedly in a thing, whether it is a higher power, your partner, yourself, or a process. Sometimes having faith in something is hard to do and people are often in a sad and lonely place when trying to renew their faith. These essential oils have been used for centuries in various rituals and ceremonies to restore and strengthen one's faith.

Essential Oils

Bergamot, cajuput, coriander, frankincense, geranium, jasmine, lavender, orange, Palo Santo, myrrh, rose, sage, and spruce

I Believe Prayer Drop

Placing one drop of lavender essential oil on the forehead has long been used to signify faith. I love to complete this ritual before meditation or prayer. The lavender helps me to focus, and I end up having so much faith in my prayers being answered that my thoughts turn into pure gratitude. Lavender is one of the few essential oils that can be applied neat. I like to apply this to my forehead, or "third eye."

Yield: 1 application

RECIPE
1 drop lavender oil

This recipe uses the direct application process whereby you can apply drops of the oils to the soles of your feet, between your eyes, your neck, or anywhere you feel you would benefit. Do not apply directly to eyes, genitals, open wounds, or mucus membranes. Store in a bottle or glass jar or a container with a tight-fitting lid in a cool, dark area for up to 3 months.

Faith in a Bottle

This blend is full of essential oils that have been reported for hundreds of years to restore faith and to bring peace and contentment to an individual. These oils have been mentioned in many religious texts concerning faith. I like to spray this in my home and in my car to restore faith in myself and others. But you can use this positivity-inducing spray just about anywhere.

Yield: 2 fluid ounces

RECIPE
4 drops spruce oil
4 drops orange oil
4 drops myrrh oil
4 drops rose oil
1 tablespoon witch hazel
2 fluid ounces water

Add all ingredients to a dark-colored spray bottle. Check for material steadfastness before spraying on fabric. Shake the bottle and spray onto area desired, such as body, hair, home, car, or office. Do not spray into or on open wounds, genitals, eyes, or mucus membranes. Store in a cool, dark area for up to 3 months. Shake well before each use to combine the ingredients.

Faith Bombs

Who says having faith has to be dull? Explode a few of these faith bombs in the bathtub and experience a whole new level of exhilaration. These oils will give you a renewed spirit of faith and joy. I love to use these bombs in the bath or shower and start my day immersing myself with my particular faith.

Yield: 12–18 bombs

RECIPE
1 cup baking soda
½ cup citric acid
½ cup cornstarch
½ cup Epsom salts, fine grained
15 drops cajuput oil
15 drops bergamot oil
10 drops Palo Santo oil

½ teaspoon carrier oil

¾ teaspoon water

spray bottle (water)

In a large bowl, mix your dry ingredients together until fine with a whisk. In a tiny jar with a lid, add your wet ingredients and shake to mix. You may add a couple drops of food coloring to the wet jar. Extremely slowly, add the wet ingredients to the dry ingredients while whisking rapidly. If fizzing takes place, whisk until it is mixed. Once the ingredients are well mixed, it should be the texture of slightly damp sand. Add a spray or two of water if needed. Once the mixture is the consistency you like, form into balls; I just smash mine down into ice cube trays or muffin tins. You can use cute molds, but you must work rapidly as mixture will dry out quickly. Leave in open air, uncovered, in a room where they will not be disturbed for 12–24 hours. Once they are dry, you can place 1–2 bombs into your bath or directly into the spray of the shower and they will fizz and release their aromatic and healing properties. Store unused portion in an airtight container for up to 6 months.

Meditation

Almost every culture has meditation of one type or another. Prayer, silence, and inward reflection are all types of meditation. There is a saying by Buddha, "You should sit in meditation for twenty minutes a day. Unless you're too busy, then you should sit for an hour." Essential oils can help to provide a feeling of relaxation, calm, and peace for that special moment for yourself each day.

Essential Oils

Cedarwood, chamomile, clary sage, frankincense, helichrysum, hyssop, lavender, and vetiver

Meditation Powder

When you put this powder under your sheets, under your meditation bolster, or under your furniture cushions, you not only set yourself up for a good night's sleep, but also meditation will come easier by calming your mind and your spirit with its antidepressant, euphoric, nervine, and sedative properties. This recipe is perfect for pondering spirituality and helping you on your path to enlightenment.

Yield: ¼ cup

RECIPE
6 drops clary sage oil
3 drops lavender oil
3 drops helichrysum oil
4 drops vitamin E oil
¼ cup cornstarch

Place the ingredients into a mason jar, stirring well with a whisk. Carefully poke holes into the lid, use this as a shaker, and shake the ingredients into pillowcases or under sheet areas as needed. You can get a piece of plastic wrap and place it over the jar and under the lid to keep powder from spilling out when not in use. Store in a glass jar or container with a tight-fitting lid in a cool, dark, and dry area for up to 3 months.

Nirvana Inhale

Carry these essential oils in a vial and use them when you need to get yourself ready for a relaxing, mind-opening session of meditation. The calming elements in these oils are euphoric, antidepressant, and tonic agents.

Yield: 1 application

RECIPE
1 drop lavender oil
or
1 drop clary sage oil
or
1 drop frankincense oil

Choose your essential oil and apply to the palm of your hand, an oil inhaler, or a tissue. Bring the essential oils close to your nostrils and inhale the aroma deeply. You can cover one nostril at a time with your thumb and, if you prefer, alternate nostrils. This process sends the properties straight to your brain and the effects are immediate. You can complete this procedure 3–4 times daily.

Meditation Air

These aromas remind me of meditation in my younger years. They automatically make me want to close my eyes and relax when I smell them. This blend contains essential oils that have nervine, hypotensive, and harmonizing properties.

Yield: 1 application

RECIPE
4 drops sandalwood oil
2 drops hyssop oil
3 drops cedarwood oil
Water

Follow your directions for using essential oils in your particular brand of diffuser. Ensure that your diffuser does not use heat but runs by vibration, sound waves, or another cold-steam type of process. Choose the essential oils needed for your condition, then add water and oils to the diffuser. Run your diffuser as needed to permeate the air with therapeutic properties and achieve the results you desire.

Mindfulness Massage

If you want a quiet massage and meditation session full of inflection and reflection, these are the essential oils to use with their sedative, antidepressant, and nervine properties.

Yield: 1 fluid ounce

RECIPE
6 drops clary sage oil
6 drops lavender oil
4 drops hyacinth oil
3 drops vitamin E oil
1 fluid ounce carrier oil

Pour the essential oils and the carrier oil into a small glass container, bowl, or jar. Swirl to mix the ingredients and use to massage lightly the area desired, such as temples, neck, chest, back, or soles of feet. Keep essential oil mixture away from open wounds, mucus membranes, genitals, eyes, and sensitive areas. Repeat application as needed. Store unused portion in a glass jar or container with a tight-fitting lid in a cool, dark area for up to 3 months.

Inflection Spritzer

This is a great spritzer to spray in your meditation room to assist getting you in the mood for a mind-altering experience while you meditate, pray, or do yoga. The mood-enhancing therapeutic properties in this blend are aphrodisiac, tranquilizing, and sedative agents.

Yield: 1 fluid ounce

RECIPE

6 drops lavender oil

5 drops frankincense oil

3 drops hyssop oil

3 drops vetiver oil

1 tablespoon witch hazel

4 fluid ounces water

Spritzers are lighter than sprays, and easier to wear on the body or in your hair. Mix the essential oils, water, and witch hazel into a spray bottle. Shake well before each use. Lightly spray the area desired, such as body, hair, clothing (check first for color damage to clothing and furniture), rooms, car, or office. The lightly scented fragrance and the healing therapeutic properties will soon make this one of your favorite methods of using your oils. Store your spritzer in a cool, dark area for up to 3 months.

Inner Light Bath Salts

Bath salts … need I say more? Meditating in the bath is one of the truly most enjoyable experiences of my life. Using these soul-refreshing essential oils while relaxing is quite peaceful and mind-expanding. This blend contains antidepressant, euphoric, hypotensive, nervine, and sedative properties.

Yield: 3 cups

RECIPE

5 drops frankincense oil

5 drops cedarwood oil

5 drops lavender oil

5 drops clary sage oil

5 drops vitamin E oil

2 tablespoons carrier oil

3 cups salts

1 tablespoon milk (optional for adults, recommended for children)

Use any type of salt you prefer: pink Himalayan salt, sea salt, Epsom salts, etc. In a small container, add the essential oils to the desired type of salt. Stir until well blended. Screw lid onto container tightly. Leave mixture in a dark area for 24 hours and then stir mixture again. Run the bathwater. Once the tub is full of water, you can add the milk, and then add ½ cup of the bath salt mixture to bathwater as you get into the tub. You may stay in the tub as long as the temperature is comfortable. Dry your feet well when you get out of the bath, as the oils are slippery and can cause you to fall. Store remainder in a glass jar or container with a tight-fitting lid in a cool, dark area for up to 3 months. These jars make attractive, inexpensive, and healing gifts!

Prayer

Prayer is that which connects us to a higher power. Every culture on earth has a form of prayer that they use to connect with their god or a higher power. Essential oils can be used to clear the mind, rid you of any negative energy, and open your soul and heart to Spirit and the universe.

Essential Oils

Angelica, cedarwood, fennel, frankincense, myrrh, rose, and sandalwood

Positive Prayer Powder

Sprinkle this under your sheets to find the right words to say when praying and open yourself up to answers from the universe. These oils have spiritually harmonizing properties. Angelica oil is very thick, but very uplifting to your soul.

Yield: ¼ cup

RECIPE

6 drops rose oil

3 drops angelica oil

3 drops cedarwood oil

4 drops vitamin E oil

¼ cup cornstarch

Place the ingredients into a mason jar, stirring well with a whisk. Carefully poke holes into the lid, use this as a shaker, and shake the ingredients into pillowcases or under sheet areas as needed. You can get a piece of plastic wrap and place it over the jar and under the lid to keep powder from spilling out when not in use. Store in a glass jar or container with a tight-fitting lid in a cool, dark, and dry area for up to 3 months.

Bless Me Bath Salts

Receive your higher power's blessings through these oils that have been used for years to open the lines of communication between you and your higher spirit. Luxuriate in this heavenly bath and use it as a time to open yourself up to communication with the divine. The only thing better than a bath with bath salts is meditating and praying while you are taking your soul-enhancing bath! This recipe contains essential oils used for thousands of years in many cultures to glorify Spirit. It's thrilling to just look at this list of ingredients.

Yield: 3 cups

RECIPE

5 drops angelica oil

5 drops myrrh oil

5 drops cedarwood oil

5 drops rose oil

4 drops vitamin E oil

2 tablespoons carrier oil

3 cups salts

1 tablespoon milk (optional for adults, recommended for children)

Use any type of salt you prefer: pink Himalayan salt, sea salt, Epsom salts, etc. In a small container, add the essential oils to the desired type of salt. Stir until well blended. Screw lid onto container tightly. Leave mixture in a dark area for 24 hours and then stir mixture again. Run the bathwater. Once the tub is full of water, you can add the milk, and then add ½ cup of the bath salt mixture to bathwater as you get into the tub. You may stay in the tub as long as the temperature is comfortable. Dry your feet well when you get out of the bath, as the oils are slippery and can cause you to fall. Store remainder in a glass jar or container with a tight-fitting lid in a cool, dark area for up to 3 months. These jars make attractive, inexpensive, and healing gifts!

Mindfully Praying

When you are devoting yourself to spending any length of time working on your soul, either through meditation, prayer, or other spirit-searching endeavors, this is the recipe that will bring you closer to Spirit and assist you with communicating your gratitude, desires, and needs.

Yield: 1 application

RECIPE

6 drops frankincense oil

4 drops myrrh oil

Water

Follow your directions for using essential oils in your particular brand of diffuser. Ensure that your diffuser does not use heat but runs by vibration, sound waves, or another cold-steam type of process. Choose the essential oils needed for your condition, then add water and oils to the diffuser. Run your diffuser as needed to permeate the air with therapeutic properties and achieve the results you desire.

Angelic Spray

The essential oils used in this spray are reported to open the pathway between us mortals and the angels above. Spray this on, and have a conversation with those above for protection and peace in your family.

Yield: 2 fluid ounces

RECIPE

7 drops angelica oil

5 drops rose oil

5 drops sandalwood oil

1 tablespoon witch hazel

2 fluid ounces water

Add all ingredients to a dark-colored spray bottle. Check for material steadfastness before spraying on fabric. Shake the bottle and spray onto area desired, such as body, hair, home, car, or office. Do not spray into or on open wounds, genitals, eyes, or mucus membranes. Store in a cool, dark area for up to 3 months. Shake well before each use to combine the ingredients.

Spiritual Spray

Opening the lines of communication between our higher power and us is sometimes not easy. Using this spray will help you to feel like you can have an open heart, spirit, and soul to pray to Spirit and share the intentions you desire, your thankfulness for what you have, and for health, health, health!

Yield: 2 fluid ounces

RECIPE

14 drops frankincense oil

9 drops myrrh oil

1 tablespoon witch hazel

2 fluid ounces water

Add all ingredients to a dark-colored spray bottle. Check for material steadfastness before spraying on fabric. Shake the bottle and spray onto area desired, such as body,

hair, home, car, or office. Do not spray into or on open wounds, genitals, eyes, or mucus membranes. Store in a cool, dark area for up to 3 months. Shake well before each use to combine the ingredients.

Heaven-Inducing Inhale

Breathing in this aroma has been used since the dawn of man to increase your ability to openly communicate with Spirit and to express that which you feel or need.

Yield: 1 application

RECIPE
1 drop angelica oil

or

1 drop myrrh oil

Choose your essential oil and apply to the palm of your hand, an oil inhaler, or a tissue. Bring the essential oils close to your nostrils and inhale the aroma deeply. You can cover one nostril at a time with your thumb and, if you prefer, alternate nostrils. This process sends the properties straight to your brain and the effects are immediate. You can complete this procedure 3–4 times daily.

Blissful Sky Bath

This bath is chock-full of the essential oils that have been used for thousands of years to help us cross that realm of selfish mortals and become the giving, loving, spiritual, grateful human beings we desire to be.

Yield: 1 application

RECIPE
6 drops cedarwood oil
6 drops sandalwood oil
1 drop fennel oil
1 tablespoon carrier oil
1 tablespoon milk (optional for adults, recommended for children)

As you begin to fill the tub with water, pour the chosen essential oils and carrier oil into the running water. Run a warm, not hot, bath. Water that is too hot will cause the essential oils to dissipate. You may add 1 tablespoon of milk to the water; this ensures that the essential oils will not stick to your skin, but will mix with the water. You may soak in the water as long as you are comfortable. Dry your feet well once you get out of the water, as the oils will cause them to be slippery, increasing your chances of falling. Rinse the tub of any remaining oils.

Spirituality

For a person to immerse themselves in dealings with the spirit and soul, essential oils can provide a perfect gateway to increase openness, calm the spirit, and remove any unwanted negative connotations. Developing your spiritual path over time is a journey full of questions, failure, wonders, and joy. Essential oils and the plants they derive from have been utilized for all of time to increase one's success on their spiritual quest. Every religion and culture on earth has used essential oils, herbs, and plants as a way to open up spiritually for a deeper connection to the Divine.

Essential Oils

Angelica, basil, bay laurel, black pepper, cassia, cinnamon, clary sage, clove, fir, frankincense, ginger, melissa, myrrh, myrtle, peppermint, pine, rosemary, scotch pine, and spruce

Spiritual Journey Powder

Sprinkle this powder under your sheets and sleep in a bed of peace and comfort knowing you are close to your higher spirit. Prayers will come easily to you and communication between you and Spirit will be clearer.

Yield: ¼ cup

RECIPE
3 drops angelica oil
3 drops frankincense oil

3 drops clary sage oil

¼ cup cornstarch

Place the ingredients into a mason jar, stirring well with a whisk. Carefully poke holes into the lid, use this as a shaker, and shake the ingredients into pillowcases or under sheet areas as needed. You can get a piece of plastic wrap and place it over the jar and under the lid to keep powder from spilling out when not in use. Store in a glass jar or container with a tight-fitting lid in a cool, dark, and dry area for up to 3 months.

The Long Path Bath Salts

Taking a spa-type meditation bath that can ground you in your faith and bring you closer to God or your Higher Spirit is a great way to build the spiritual base you crave. These essential oils are a perfect way to continue your journey of enlightenment.

Yield: 3 cups

RECIPE

5 drops rosemary oil

5 drops clary sage oil

5 drops melissa oil

5 drops ginger oil

2 tablespoons carrier oil

3 cups salts

1 tablespoon milk (optional for adults, recommended for children)

Use any type of salt you prefer: pink Himalayan salt, sea salt, Epsom salts, etc. In a small container, add the essential oils to the desired type of salt. Stir until well blended. Screw lid onto container tightly. Leave mixture in a dark area for 24 hours and then stir mixture again. Run the bathwater. Once the tub is full of water, you can add the milk, and then add ½ cup of the bath salt mixture to bathwater as you get into the tub. You may stay in the tub as long as the temperature is comfortable. Dry your feet well when you get out of the bath, as the oils are slippery and can cause you to fall. Store remainder in a glass jar or container with a tight-fitting lid in a cool, dark area for up to 3 months. These jars make attractive, inexpensive, and healing gifts!

Mala Inhale

When entering a place of worship or beginning meditation or prayer, these are the aromas you want to inhale—try it with mala beads! Taking a whiff of these essential oils gets my mind, my soul, and heart synchronized and in the spirit of praying.

Yield: 1 application

RECIPE
1 drop frankincense oil
or
1 drop angelica oil
or
1 drop clary sage oil

Choose your essential oil and apply to the palm of your hand, an oil inhaler, or a tissue. Bring the essential oils close to your nostrils and inhale the aroma deeply. You can cover one nostril at a time with your thumb and, if you prefer, alternate nostrils. This process sends the properties straight to your brain and the effects are immediate. You can complete this procedure 3–4 times daily.

Angelic Cloud

This diffuser recipe is said to connect one with those who have passed. It is a comforting and warm recipe that works well when used in times of reflection.

Yield: 1 application

RECIPE
3 drops ginger oil
3 drops melissa oil
3 drops pine oil
Water

Follow your directions for using essential oils in your particular brand of diffuser. Ensure that your diffuser does not use heat but runs by vibration, sound waves, or another cold-steam type of process. Choose the essential oils needed for your condition, then add water and oils to the diffuser. Run your diffuser as needed to permeate the air with therapeutic properties and achieve the results you desire.

Hallowed Bath

This bath uses essential oils that have long been purported to open thinking and prayer when communing with Higher Spirit. Open your mind and heart while relaxing in these peaceful and calming scents.

Yield: 1 application

RECIPE
4 drops angelica oil
3 drops frankincense oil
3 drops myrrh oil
1 tablespoon carrier oil
1 tablespoon milk (optional for adults, recommended for children)

As you begin to fill the tub with water, pour the chosen essential oils and carrier oil into the running water. Run a warm, not hot, bath. Water that is too hot will cause the essential oils to dissipate. You may add 1 tablespoon of milk to the water; this ensures that the essential oils will not stick to your skin, but will mix with the water. You may soak in the water as long as you are comfortable. Dry your feet well once you get out of the water, as the oils will cause them to be slippery, increasing your chances of falling. Rinse the tub of any remaining oils.

Worship

There are so many types of worship in our world today. No matter what religion you are, worship means to have unquestioning reverence for a higher power. You can worship through prayer, thoughts, acts, and religious rites. Essential oils have been used for thousands of years as a means of expressing adoration and worship in every culture on earth.

Essential Oils

Angelica, cedarwood, clary sage, frankincense, geranium, lemon, lotus, melissa, myrrh, rosemary, sandalwood, and wild orange

I Surrender

These aromas wafting through the air bring a sense of peace and honor and can help one to venerate their higher power. Use this when going into a time of meditation or prayer. These oils will help to open your mind, gather your thoughts, and communicate more effectively.

Yield: 1 application

RECIPE
3 drops melissa oil
2 drops wild orange oil
2 drops myrrh oil
Water

Follow your directions for using essential oils in your particular brand of diffuser. Ensure that your diffuser does not use heat but runs by vibration, sound waves, or another cold-steam type of process. Choose the essential oils needed for your condition, then add water and oils to the diffuser. Run your diffuser as needed to permeate the air with therapeutic properties and achieve the results you desire.

Blessed Ointment

This ointment contains some of the holiest of essential oils to help bring honor and respect to a situation or religious rite. These oils have been used throughout history as a means to express gratitude and surrender to Spirit.

Yield: 1 tablespoon

RECIPE
3 teaspoons carrier oil
½ teaspoon beeswax pellets
4 drops vitamin E oil

2 drops frankincense oil

2 drops lemon oil

2 drops clary sage oil

Heat the beeswax and the carrier oil in a glass bowl in the microwave for 1 ½–2 minutes, until just melted, or on low on the stove top. If you open the door every 15 seconds, you can avoid the popping of the wax and oil and overheating. Carefully remove the container from the microwave and stir. Drip a drop of the melted oil and wax onto the counter, after 1 minute check for consistency. If it is too thin, add more beeswax to the container; if it is too thick, add more carrier oil. Add the vitamin E oil and the essential oil to the heated mixture in the container. Whisk lightly, and it will begin hardening immediately. Pour into containers. Ensure your containers are glass or tin to prevent leeching of chemicals. Once cool, apply to wrists, temples, neck, or soles of feet. Do not apply to mucus membranes, eyes, genitals, or open wounds. Label containers and store in a dark, dry area for up to 1 year.

Glorifying Spray

This recipe contains a blend of essential oils that are often used together to promote reverence and honor to a higher power. I can be used in a room where several people are gathering to show their respect with praise and worship or meditate.

Yield: 2 fluid ounces

RECIPE

9 drops sandalwood oil

5 drops myrrh oil

5 drops melissa oil

1 tablespoon witch hazel

2 fluid ounces water

Add all ingredients to a dark-colored spray bottle. Check for material steadfastness before spraying on fabric. Shake the bottle and spray onto area desired, such as body, hair, home, car, or office. Do not spray into or on open wounds, genitals, eyes, or mucus membranes. Store in a cool, dark area for up to 3 months. Shake well before each use to combine the ingredients.

Conclusion

Essential oils can play a huge part in our daily quest for assistance with our conditions, emotions, needs, desires, and devotions. Learning how to use essential oils, heed warnings, store the oils, and differentiate between various healing methods can be extremely beneficial for every aspect of our lives.

Even though essential oils have been used by every culture on earth for thousands of years, using oils may be new to you. Through the use of this book, you can absorb knowledge of these oils easily and rapidly. Access to essential oils that are wholesome, safe, and ethically produced is now readily available to anyone. Learning to apply and use the oils the right way can improve your life dramatically in so many ways.

My fervent desire is that you have used, learned, and felt the healing and empowering benefits of essential oils after reading this book. I know the multitude of life enhancements I have received from these recipes, and I want the same for you. Above all, don't be afraid to use your oils. They are from the earth. They were made for you.

Acknowledgments

I wish to first thank my family for always being the most supportive people ever. I don't know how I got so lucky to have the family that I do. All of you are at the top of my brain at all times. Unceasingly. I'm a lucky, lucky girl!

My daughters, Lin and Colleen—you girls! You have had more faith in me than I have ever had in myself. You both have been such an instrumental part in everything I have ever done. Your words (I mean shouts!) of encouragement mean more to me than you will ever know. You are, and always have been, the best daughters a mother could ever wish for. I love your company and will happily live with you both when I get old. You can take turns. Go us!

I would like to take the time to give a special thank you to my sister, Michele McDaniel. Chele, I don't know where I would be in this world without you. You are the most honest, wise, and beautiful woman that I know. You always know what to say to make me feel better, and you know when to egg me on when I need it. We have been together through it all. You are the person I turn to with every little heartache and every tiny joy. I love you so much and can't imagine my world without you in it. You are the biggest blessing in my life and in the lives of so many others. We all thank God for you every day. Beanie Weanie, Chele!

To my brother, Mike. We are about as different as two people can possibly be. Our greatest strength is to just "agree to disagree." You are the funniest person I know, and no one can make me laugh like you do. I love you, I would die for you, and above all, I respect you. Thank you for loving me, Mike. I love you so much, brother.

I want to thank all of my team at Llewellyn for their tireless revisions and the great communication about my book. That art department is the bomb! I want to give a special shout out to Brian Erdrich and Angela Wix. They made me feel like they were devoted to my book and my desires above all else. You guys are the rock stars of all the editors in the world. My gratitude to you runs deep.

I want to thank Murphy Rae (Indie Solutions) for her initial editing of this book. Her insight was valuable and I love her so much. Hi, Asher!

My agent is Jane Dystel of Dystel and Goderich. Need I say more? Her reputation precedes her for a reason…she gets sh*t done! Thank you, Jane, for your devotion to your clients and your ability to "read between the lines (and words)." I am forever indebted to you and your brilliance in this publishing world.

Thank you to Miriam Goderich for stepping in when needed. What a powerhouse duo the two of you are. My gratitude is boundless.

My husband, Vance. You are the glue, mister, and we all love you so much more than you will ever know or believe. I hope when you get to heaven that there is time travel, and you will get to spend eternity in the 1800s fishing, hunting, and living in a tent. I really like the 2000s, but I will live in the 1800s if I get to live with you. But I ain't gonna chew on any leather to make you a soft blanket. You can get over that dream. I love you beyond eternity.

To my mom and dad, Vannoy Gentles and Tom Gentles. My biggest supporters. I live to make you guys proud of me. This book was written with a lot of time taken away from both of you, but y'all never complained. I love you both so very much. I hope that your future, with us kids, is full of the joy and happiness that you both so truly deserve. Everything I have, I owe to both of you. I love you and want to do any and everything in my power to bring some "gold" to your golden years. I wish you peace and love.

To my friends. I know that I get caught up in writing these books, the yoga studio, the store, life, and I put everything, including you, on the back burner. I am a horrible friend. I know that. I am the worst. I hate plans. I hate talking on the phone. I don't like to go anywhere. I'm always busy with family, work, and projects. Yet you all still support me, talk to me, and love me. I adore you all very, very much; more than you can imagine. Theresa, Teena, Angela, Tina, Betsy, Donna, Maria, Rosa, Terisa, Patricia—you guys are the BFFs of all BFFs. No matter how long we go without seeing each other, we can always pick it up like there was no separation at all. I thank you so much for hanging in there with me, always supporting me, encouraging me, soliciting my advice (when I really never know what I'm talking about), and giving me advice when I am manic. Someday I will be a good friend and call you and make a plan. This is a plan … to someday make a plan. I call that progress in the friendship department. Cruise 2020 … there! An actual plan! Go Me!

To everyone who buys and uses this book. Thank you! I love you all and pray that you find solace, comfort, and healing throughout the thousands of times you will use this book. It is for *you* I write, research, and continue on this winding path. Your support, emails, cards, messages, critiques, letters, feedback, reviews, and gifts mean the world to me—more than you will ever know. I hope you have a lifetime of spiritual and emotional peace and fulfillment.

To my Yogis … I love you. I love you. I love you … breathe.

Glossary of Technical Terms

I have listed some of the most common technical terms used in this book. Become familiar with the most common terms, as learning these definitions of the technical terms will give you the knowledge of how to use new essential oils in the future for your own recipes. Essential oils have more than one therapeutic property and each oil can help to heal a wide variety of ailments. Knowing what these terms mean can bring a whole world of healing and usage to you and/or your family.

Analgesic: Lowers pain

Anti-allergenic: Assists in lowering allergy symptoms

Antibacterial: Destroys bacteria and reduces the ability of bacteria to reproduce

Antibiotic: Assists in fighting bacterial infections

Anti-carcinogenic: Contains cancer-fighting properties

Anticatarrhal: Removes excess mucus in the body, assists with respiratory ailments

Antidepressant: Assists in alleviating depression

Antiemetic: Soothes upset stomach, relieves nausea and vomiting

Antifungal: Assists in relieving fungal attacks, itching, and spreading

Anti-infectious: Fights against infection

Anti-inflammatory: Relieves inflamed areas, cools

Antimicrobial: Stops the growth of microorganisms

Antiparasitic: Used to treat parasitic diseases

Antiphlogistic: Reduces redness and inflammation

Antirheumatic: Reduces arthritis pain and swelling

Antiseptic: Cleans and is used in fighting germs and infections

Antispasmodic: Reduces spasms and cramping

Antitussive: Relieves coughs and respiratory ailments

Antivenous: Prevents blood clots

Antiviral: Used to treat viral infections

Aperient: Helps to relieve constipation

Aphrodisiac: Increases sexual desire

Aromatic: Imparts a pleasing aroma

Astringent: Helps to tighten the skin

Bactericidal: Kills living bacteria

Balsamic: Has balsam oil in the ingredients

Carminative: Relieves bloating and gas

Cephalic: Relates to head injuries and illness

Cholagogue: Promotes discharge and flow of bile

Cicatrisant: Used for cell regeneration, heals scars

Circulatory stimulant: Promotes blood circulation

Cordial: Warm and comforting, imparts good feelings

Cytophylactic: Beneficial for aging and mature skin

Decongestant: Thins and reduces mucus

Depurative: Helps to rid the digestive system of waste and toxins

Detoxifying: Used to remove toxins and poisons from the body

Diaphoretic: Helps rid the body of toxins through perspiration

Diuretic: Induces the flow of urine to rid the body of water and bloating

Emmenagogue: Induces menstruation

Emollient: Produces a softening and smoothing of the skin

Euphoric: Brings a sense of extreme pleasure

Expectorant: Helps the lungs and respiratory system rid the body of excess mucus

Febrifuge: Used to help reduce a fever

Fungicidal: Inhibits the growth of fungus

Galactogogue: Helps to promote lactating in women

Haemostatic: Stops the flow of blood

Hepatic: Used to promote liver function

Hypertensive: Lowers blood pressure

Hypotensive: Raises blood pressure

Lymphatic: Relates to lymph secretions

Mucolytic: Sedative used to help to break down mucus

Nervine: Calms and soothes nervous system

Ophthalmic: Beneficial for the eyes

Rubefacient: Causes skin to redden by increasing blood flow

Sedative: Calming, soothing, tranquilizing

Stomachic: Helps to increase appetite

Styptic: Used to stop the flow of blood from a wound

Sudorific: Causes increased perspiration

Tonic: Promotes a feeling of well-being and increased vitality

Vasodilator: Opens the blood vessels for increased circulation

Vermifuge: Used to kill and treat parasites

Vulnerary: Used to heal wounds and prevent infection

Warnings for Each Essential Oil

*E*ssential oils can be the most healing product in the world... or the most harmful. You must visit your doctor to ensure that essential oils won't compromise any medications you are currently taking or any conditions you may have. Perform a patch test on yourself or your loved one to ensure no allergies to any essential oils are present. I am not a doctor, nor am I a diagnostician. Below are a few of the warnings I found to be pertinent with most of the essential oils used in this book. This is by no means a complete list of the warnings and contraindications of each essential oil. Always complete a patch test on yourself or your loved one before using an essential oil and watch for adverse reactions. How to complete a patch test is explained in the "But First: Tips and Warnings" section of this book. I may indicate when I didn't come across warnings, but that doesn't mean there aren't any. Please complete your own research about using essential oils with your condition or ailment and medications.

Warnings

Aloe Vera Oil
No warnings discovered by this author.

Agrimony Oil

Prolonged usage can lead to stomach issues. Agrimony can increase allergies in some people.

Amber Oil

Do not use if you are pregnant, nursing, or think you may be pregnant.

Angelica Oil

Do not use if you are pregnant, nursing, or think you may be pregnant. Do not use if you have diabetes, epilepsy, or seizures, or on children. This oil is phototoxic, and therefore should not be used before prolonged sun exposure.

Anise Oil

Anise oil should not be used for prolonged periods of time. Do not use if you are pregnant, nursing, or think you may be pregnant.

Arnica Oil

Arnica oil should never be taken internally or applied to an open wound. Always use a carrier oil with arnica oil. A patch test should be used with arnica oil as it is known for causing skin issues and allergies in certain people.

Balsam Oil

Balsam oil is one of the most allergy-producing substances on earth. Ensure that you are not allergic by performing a patch test. Prolonged usage is not advisable.

Basil Oil

Always use a carrier oil with basil oil as it can burn the skin. Do not use in bathwater as it can burn the skin. Do not use if you have epilepsy, seizures, or are pregnant, nursing, or think you may be pregnant.

Bay Oil

Use sparingly for short durations of time. Do not use if you are pregnant, nursing, or think you may be pregnant.

Benzoin

Should not be used in bathwater or in a diffuser as it is very thick and sticky and will adhere to skin. Always use a carrier oil to help dilute the benzoin. Do not use on children.

Bergamot Oil

Do not use if you are pregnant, nursing, or think you may be pregnant. This oil is phototoxic, and therefore should not be used before prolonged sun exposure. Always dilute with a carrier oil before applying topically.

Birch Oil

Birch oil is very potent. Always dilute with a carrier oil before applying topically. Birch oil has had some severe allergies associated with its usage. Ensure you are not suffering any side effects with a patch test before using birch oil. Do not use if you are pregnant, nursing, or think you may be pregnant.

Black Pepper Oil

Do not use black pepper oil if you have any kidney issues as it can cause kidney damage.

Blue Chamomile Oil

(See Chamomile Oil)

Blue Cypress Oil

(See Cypress Oil)

Borage Seed Oil

Borage seed oil can cause thinning of the blood. Do not take if you have upcoming tattoos or surgeries. Do not take borage seed oil if you have any liver issues.

Cajuput Oil

Please check with your physician before beginning a regimen of mixing cajuput oil with other medications. Do not use on children.

Calendula Oil

Do not use if you are pregnant, nursing, or think you may be pregnant.

Camphor Oil

Do not use on open wounds or mucus membranes. Do not heat camphor oil or use on children.

Cardamom Oil

Always conduct a patch test before beginning a new oil. Cardamom has caused skin issues in some people.

Cassia Oil

Cassia oil should always be mixed with a carrier oil before usage as it can cause burns due to its potency.

Cedarwood Oil

Do not use on children. Cedarwood oil can terminate a pregnancy. Do not use if you are pregnant, nursing, or think you may be pregnant or are trying to conceive.

Chamomile Oil

Chamomile oil can irritate the skin. Do not use if you are pregnant, nursing, or think you may be pregnant.

Cilantro Oil

No warnings discovered by this author.

Cinnamon Bark Oil

Cinnamon bark oil should not be used by those undergoing cancer treatments such as chemotherapy or radiation. This oil should always be diluted with a carrier oil as it can cause significant burns to the skin if undiluted. Do not use if you are pregnant, nursing, or think you may be pregnant.

Citrus Oils

These oils are phototoxic, and therefore should not be used before prolonged sun exposure.

Clary Sage Oil

Do not use if you have low blood pressure, or if you are hypoglycemic. Can cause drowsiness, so it's better to not drive or operate heavy machinery while using this oil. Do not use if you are pregnant, trying to get pregnant, nursing, or think you may be pregnant.

Clematis Oil

Can cause skin irritations if applied without dilution.

Clove Oil

A natural blood thinner, do not take if you are taking blood thinners or are scheduled for an upcoming tattoo or surgery. Clove oil is very thick and strong, do not use in diffuser or in baths. Always dilute with a carrier oil. Do not use if you are pregnant, nursing, or think you may be pregnant.

Comfrey Oil

Do not take internally. Do not take if you have a liver disease, or a serious disease such as cancer. Do not use if you are pregnant, nursing, or think you may be pregnant.

Coriander Oil

Do not take if you have any kidney issues or if you are pregnant, nursing, or think you may be pregnant.

Cosmos Oil

No warnings discovered by this author.

Cypress Oil

Do not use if you are pregnant, nursing, or think you may be pregnant.

Dill Oil

No warnings discovered by this author.

Echinacea Oil

No warnings discovered by this author.

Eucalyptus Oil

Eucalyptus can trigger asthma attacks, and should never be used in conjunction with other medications, on the face, on children, or by persons with high blood pressure.

Fennel Oil

Fennel oil should not be used if you have a disorder such as seizures, cancer, kidney issues, or hormone problems. Do not use if you are pregnant, nursing, or think you may be pregnant.

Fir Oil

Do not use if you are pregnant, nursing, or think you may be pregnant.

Frankincense Oil

Do not use if you are pregnant, nursing, or think you may be pregnant, especially during the first trimester of pregnancy.

Garlic Oil

Do not give garlic oil to babies. Do not use if you are pregnant, nursing, or think you may be pregnant.

Geranium Oil

Do not use if you are pregnant, nursing, or think you may be pregnant. Do not use if you have low blood sugar or have skin issues. May cause insomnia.

German Chamomile Oil

(See Chamomile Oil)

Ginger Oil

Do not use ginger oil if you are on blood thinners, have sensitive skin, or have gallstones.

Ginkgo Biloba Oil

No warnings discovered by this author.

Ginseng Oil

No warnings discovered by this author.

Grapefruit Oil

This oil is phototoxic, and therefore should not be used before prolonged sun exposure. Do not use if you have a skin condition as it can irritate the skin.

Helichrysum Oil (Immortelle, everlasting)

Do not use with blood thinners or with children. Do not use if you are pregnant, nursing, or think you may be pregnant.

Hibiscus Oil

Do not use if you are pregnant, nursing, or think you may be pregnant.

Holly Oil

No warnings discovered by this author.

Honeysuckle Oil

No warnings discovered by this author.

Hyssop Oil

Do not use if you are pregnant, nursing, or think you may be pregnant. Do not use if you suffer from a seizure disorder or high blood pressure. Do not mix with other medications.

Jasmine Oil

Do not use if you are pregnant, nursing, or think you may be pregnant.

Juniper Berry Oil

Do not take for extended periods of time. Do not take if you have kidney issues. Do not mix with other medications. Do not use if you are pregnant, nursing, or think you may be pregnant.

Lavender Oil

No warnings discovered by this author.

Lemon Oil

This oil is phototoxic, and therefore should not be used before prolonged sun exposure. Do not use if you are pregnant, nursing, or think you may be pregnant. Can cause skin irritation.

Lemon Balm Oil (Melissa)

Do not take if you have thyroid issues. Do not use if you are pregnant, nursing, or think you may be pregnant. May cause drowsiness.

Lemongrass Oil

Do not use if you are pregnant, nursing, or think you may be pregnant.

Lemon Thyme Oil

Do not use if you are pregnant, nursing, or think you may be pregnant.

Lime Oil

Do not use if you are pregnant, nursing, or think you may be pregnant. This oil is phototoxic, and therefore should not be used before prolonged sun exposure.

Linden Blossom Oil

No warnings discovered by this author.

Lotus Oil

Not enough known about use during pregnancy. Avoid if pregnant or nursing. No other warnings discovered by this author.

Mandarin Oil

This oil is phototoxic, and therefore should not be used before prolonged sun exposure.

Manuka Oil

No warnings discovered by this author.

Marjoram Oil

Do not use if you are taking blood thinners, or suffer from depression. Do not use if you are pregnant, nursing, or think you may be pregnant.

Melaleuca Oil

(See Tea Tree Oil)

Melissa Oil (Lemon balm oil)

Do not take if you have thyroid issues. Do not use if you are pregnant, nursing, or think you may be pregnant. May cause drowsiness.

Myrrh Oil

Do not use if you are pregnant, nursing, or think you may be pregnant.

Myrtle Oil

Do not use internally or with children or any pulmonary issues. Do not use if you are pregnant, nursing, or think you may be pregnant.

Neem Oil

Do not use internally or with children or any pulmonary issues. Do not use if you are pregnant, nursing, or think you may be pregnant. Do not use if you have autoimmune disorders, have multiple sclerosis or rheumatoid arthritis, or suffer from any liver issues.

Neroli Oil

Neroli can be a skin irritant in some people. Do not use on children.

Niaouli Oil

No warnings discovered by this author.

Orange Oil

This oil is phototoxic, and therefore should not be used before prolonged sun exposure.

Oregano Oil

Do not apply directly to skin, such as in the bathtub, as it can cause rashes or burns on skin. Always dilute oregano oil with a carrier oil. Do not use if you are pregnant, nursing, or think you may be pregnant.

Oregon Grape root Oil

Do not use if you are pregnant, nursing, or think you may be pregnant.

Palmarosa Oil

No warnings discovered by this author.

Patchouli Oil

Patchouli oil should not be ingested by persons with any eating disorders.

Peppermint Oil

Peppermint oil can cause skin irritation, so do not use in the bath. Never use peppermint oil with prescribed medications. Do not use if you are pregnant, nursing, or think you may be pregnant.

Peru Balsam Oil

Do not use if you are pregnant, nursing, or think you may be pregnant. Do not use if you suffer from allergies, or kidney issues. Do not take internally.

Petitgrain Oil

No warnings discovered by this author.

Pine Oil

Do not use if you have sensitive skin as pine oil can irritate skin. Do not use if you have high blood pressure. Do not use if you are pregnant, nursing, or think you may be pregnant.

Pink Grapefruit Oil

No warnings discovered by this author.

Poppy Oil

No warnings discovered by this author.

Ravensara Oil

No warnings discovered by this author.

Roman Chamomile Oil

Chamomile oil can irritate the skin. Do not use if you are pregnant, nursing, or think you may be pregnant.

Rose Oil

Do not use if you are pregnant, nursing, or think you may be pregnant.

Rosemary Oil

Do not use if you have seizures, high blood pressure, epilepsy, or are trying to get pregnant. Do not use if you are pregnant, nursing, or think you may be pregnant. Do not use on children.

Sage Oil

Not safe to use if you suffer from high blood pressure or any type of seizures.

Sandalwood Oil

Do not use if you have any kidney issues. Can cause allergic skin reactions, so a patch test should be completed before using.

Sesame Oil

No warnings discovered by this author.

Spearmint Oil

Do not take internally. Do not use if you are pregnant, nursing, or think you may be pregnant.

Spikenard Oil

Do not use if you are pregnant, nursing, or think you may be pregnant.

Spruce Oil

Do not use if you are pregnant, nursing, or think you may be pregnant. Do not take if you suffer from any type of heart condition or asthma.

St. John's Wort Oil

Do not mix with other medications unless under supervision of your prescribing doctor. Watch for side effects. Perform a patch test before using. This oil is phototoxic, and therefore should not be used before prolonged sun exposure.

Sweet Orange Oil

Use caution when giving to children and do not use for long periods of time. This oil is phototoxic, and therefore should not be used before prolonged sun exposure.

Tangerine Oil

This oil is phototoxic, and therefore should not be used before prolonged sun exposure.

Tarragon Oil

Do not use if you are pregnant, nursing, or think you may be pregnant.

Tea Tree Oil

No warnings discovered by this author.

Thyme Oil

Do not use in the bathtub as it will cling to skin and burn. This oil is too thick to use in a diffuser and my harm your diffuser. Do not use on children. Do not use if you have high blood pressure. Do not use if you are pregnant, nursing, or think you may be pregnant.

Trumpet Vine Oil

No warnings discovered by this author.

Valerian Oil

This oil does not have enough evidence to present as safe to use during pregnancy or breastfeeding or trying to conceive. I would advise to not use during those times. Do not combine with other medications.

Vanilla Oil

No warnings discovered by this author.

Vetiver Oil

Do not take consistently for long periods of time.

Vitamin E Oil

Do not ingest internally.

Wheat Germ Oil

No warnings discovered by this author. Please complete your own research before using this oil. Do not use if you are a celiac.

White Fir Oil

No warnings discovered by this author.

Wild Orange Oil

No warnings discovered by this author.

Wintergreen Oil

There are many warnings about wintergreen oil. It is a very effective arthritis pain reliever, but do not use for extended periods of time. Ensure through your physician that it is safe to use wintergreen oil with your prescribed medications. Watch for side effects. Do not give to children. Do not use if you are pregnant, nursing, or think you may be pregnant.

Yarrow Oil

Has been known to cause headaches in some people. Do not use if you are pregnant, nursing, or think you may be pregnant.

Ylang-Ylang Oil

Do not use if you are on blood thinners or have high blood pressure. May cause headaches, watch for side effects. Can cause skin allergies in some people. Do not use if you are pregnant, nursing, or think you may be pregnant.

APPENDIX 2
Therapeutic Properties of Each Essential Oil

*E*very plant, shrub, herb, tree, flower, fruit, and vegetable on earth contains therapeutic properties. Scientists have worked diligently for the last century to find out what those properties are and how they can be manipulated, copied, extracted, and used for disease and health.

Pharmaceutical companies copy the natural chemical compounds that make up the therapeutic properties from plants and develop chemically based substitutes to be made into medicines. The chemical copies are cheaper and easier to regulate, produce, and distribute than the production of plants and natural medicines would be, but they often aren't as useful for the body. Americans pay billions of dollars to pharmaceutical companies annually for the chemical copies of plants.

Below is a list of the most commonly used essential oils and a few of their therapeutic properties. We can thank science for giving us these technical terms, but actually, our ancestors have been using these plants for thousands of years for these very same healing and spiritual purposes.

Therapeutic Properties

Agrimony (*Agrimonia eupatoria*)

Antianxiety, anti-inflammatory, antioxidant, digestive, diuretic

Aloe Vera (*Aloe Barbadensis Miller*)

Analgesic, antibacterial, antifungal, anti-inflammatory, anti-irritant, antioxidant, antiviral, astringent, cicatrisant, cytophylactic, diuretic, emollient, vulnerary

Amber (*Pinus Succinfera*)

Analgesic, anti-inflammatory, antispasmodic, aphrodisiac, aromatic, calming, pain reliever, respiratory, rheumatoid

Angelica (*Angelica Archangelica*)

Antispasmodic, carminative, depurative, diaphoretic, digestive, diuretic, emenagogue, expectorant, febrifuge, hepatic, holy, nervine, ritualistic, stimulant, stomachic, tonic

Anise (*Pimpinella Anisum*)

Anti-epileptic, anti-hysteric, antirheumatic, antiseptic, anti-spasmodic, aperient, carminative, cordial, culinary, decongestant, digestive, expectorant, insecticide, respiratory, sedative, stimulant, vermifuge

Balsam (*Myroxylon Balsamum*)

Allergies, antibacterial, anti-inflammatory, antioxidant, antiseptic, cicatrisant, deodorant, diuretic, expectorant

Basil (*Ocimum basilicum*)

Analgesic, culinary, antibacterial, antibiotic, antidepressant, immune boosting, antifungal, anti-infectious, anti-inflammatory, antiseptic, anti-spasmodic, antiviral, calming, carminative, digestive tonic, earaches, emenagogue, holy, intestinal, intestinal, ophthalmic, relaxant, restorative, rituals, stimulant, stomachic

Bay Laurel (*Laurus nobilis*)

Analgesic, aromatic, emetic, emmenagogue, nervine, rheumatoid, stimulant

Benzoin (*Lindera Benzoin*)

Analgesic, antidepressant, anti-inflammatory, antirheumatic, antiseptic, astringent, carminative, cordial, deodorant, disinfectant, diuretic, euphoric, expectorant, relaxant, sedative, vulnerary, warming

Bergamot (*Citrus Bergamia*)

Analgesic, antianxiety, antibiotic, antidepressant, antiseptic, antispasmodic, aromatic, cicatrisant, deodorant, digestive, disinfectant, febrifuge, vermifuge, vulnerary, weight reduction, uplifting

Birch (*Betula Alba*)

Analgesic, aromatic, antiarthritic, antidepressant, cicatrisant, antibacterial, antifungal, anti-inflammatory, antirheumatic, antiarthritic, antiseptic, antispasmodic, astringent, disinfectant, depurative, diuretic, febrifuge, germicide, insecticide, tonic, stimulant, detoxifier

Black Pepper (*Piper Nigrum*)

Analgesic, antiarthritic, antibacterial, anticatarrhal, anti-inflammatory, antioxidant, antirheumatic, antiseptic, anti-spasmodic, aperient, carminative, culinary, diaphoretic, digestive, expectorant, respiratory, warming

Blue Cypress (*Callitris Intratropica*)

Antibacterial, anti-inflammatory, antirheumatic, soothing, warming

Borage Seed (*Borago Officinalis*)

Antiarthritic, anticatarrhal, antidepressant, anti-inflammatory, antirheumatic, antiulcer, cicatrisant, diuretic, demulcent, emollient, febrifuge, hormonal, purifier

Cajeput (*Melaleuca Leucadendra*)

Analgesic, antifungal, antineuralgic, antioxidant, antiseptic, antispasmodic, bactericide, carminative, cosmetic, decongestant, diaphoretic, emenagogue, expectorant, febrifuge, insecticide, respiratory, stimulant, sudorific, tonic, vermifuge, vulnerary

Calendula (*Pot marigold/Tagetes Glandulifera*)

Antibruising, anticarcinogenic, anti-inflammatory, anti-itch, antipyretic, antispasmodic, antiulcer, carminative, cicatrisant, emenagogue, menstrual cramps, sudorific, tonic, vulnerary

Camphor (*Cinnamoman Camphora*)

Anesthetic, antianxiety, anti-inflammatory, antineuralgic, antiseptic, antispasmodic, decongestant, disinfectant, insecticide, nervine, sedative

Cardamom (*Elettaria Cardamomum*)

Antimicrobial, carminative, antiseptic, antispasmodic, antioxidant, aphrodisiac, astringent, carminative, digestive, diuretic, expectorant, stimulant, stomachic

Carrot Seed (*Daucus Carota*)

Antiseptic, carminative, cytophylactic, depurative, detoxifying, diuretic, emenagogue, tonic, vermifuge

Cassia (*Cinnamonum Cassia*)

Antiarthritic, anti-diarrheal, antidepressant, antiemetic, antigalactogogue, antimicrobial, antirheumatic, antiviral, aromatic, astringent, carminative, circulatory, culinary, digestive, emenagogue, febrifuge, immune booster, stimulant, uplifting, warming

Cedarwood (*Cedrus Atlantica*)

Antirheumatic, antiseborrhoeic, antispasmodic, aromatic, astringent, comforting, digestive, diuretic, emmenagogue, expectorant, fungicide, grounding, insecticidal, sedative, tonic

Chamomile (*Matricaria Chamomilla*)

Analgesic, aromatic, antiallergenic, antibiotic, antidepressant, antifungal, anti-infectious, comforting, anti-inflammatory, antimicrobial, antineuralgic, antiphlogistic, antiseptic, antispasmodic, bactericidal, carminative, cholagogue, cicatrisant, cooling, deodorant, digestive, emmenagogue, febrifuge, hepatic, nervine, sedative, sudorific, stomachic, tonic, vermifuge, vulnerary, warming

- **German** *(Matricaria Recutita)* Analgesic, anti-allergenic, antibacterial, anticatarrhal, anti-inflammatory, antiseptic, antispasmodic, carminative, digestive, fungicidal, nervine, sedative
- **Roman** *(Anthemus Nobilis)* Anti-inflammatory, antibiotic, antidiuretic, antimicrobial, antineuralgic, antiphlogistic, antiseptic, antispasmodic, antitumor, aromatic, bactericidal, carminative, cholagogue, digestive, hepatic, sedative, tonic

Cinnamon (*Cinnamomum Zeylanicum*)

Analgesic, antibacterial, anticarcinogenic, anticlotting, antifungal, antimicrobial, antioxidant, aromatic, astringent, carminative, cooling, culinary, digestive, hypotensive, insecticide, stimulating, uplifting

Citrus (*Citron*)

Antibacterial, antitoxic, antiviral, aromatic, astringent, circulatory, culinary, detoxifying, germicidal, uplifting

Clary Sage (*Salvia Sclarea*)

Anticonvulsive, antidepressant, antispasmodic, aphrodisiac, aromatic, astringent, bactericidal, calming, carminative, deodorant, digestive, emenagogue, euphoric, hormones, hypotensive, nervine, ophthalmic, perfumery, sedative, soothing, stomachic, tonic, uterine vulnerary

Clematis (*Clematis Alpena*)

Antispasmodic, antisyphilis, antiulcer, cicatrisant, nervine, stomachic, varicose veins, vulnerary

Clove (*Syzygium Aromaticum*)

Analgesic, anesthetic, antifungal, anti-inflammatory, antimicrobial, antirheumatic, antiseptic, antiviral, aphrodisiac, aromatic, bactericidal, carminative, culinary, insecticide, stimulant

Comfrey (*Symphytum*)

Antibronchitis, anti-inflammatory, antirheumatic, antiulcer, diarrhea, heavy menstrual periods, respiratory, vulnerary

Coriander (*Coriandrum Sativum*)

Analgesic, antirheumatic, antispasmodic, aphrodisiac, aromatic, carminative, culinary, deodorant, depurative, diarrhea, flatulence, hemorrhoids, hernia, lipolytic, nausea, stimulant, stomachic

Cosmos (*Cosmos Bipinnatus*)

Antibacterial, antioxidant, aromatic, insecticidal

Cypress (*Cupressus Sempervirens*)

Anti-infectious, anti-inflammatory, antiparasitic, antirheumatic, antiseptic, antispasmodic, astringent, decongestant, deodorant, diuretic, restorative, vasoconstrictor

Dill (*Anethum Graveolens*)

Antiarthritic, antispasmodic, antimicrobial, antioxidant, carminative, culinary, digestive, disinfectant, galactogogue, sedative, stomachic, sudorific

Echinacea (*Echinacea Purpurea*)

Analgesic, anti-allergen, antibacterial, antibiotic, anti-infectious, anti-inflammatory, antioxidant, immune booster, respiratory

Eucalyptus (*Eucalyptus Globulus*)

Analgesic, antibacterial, antifungal, anti-inflammatory, antimicrobial, antiseptic, antispasmodic, antiviral, aromatic, bactericidal, decongestant, deodorant, diuretic, expectorant, mucolytic, stimulating, tonic vulnerary

Fennel (*Foeniculum vulgare*)

Analgesic, antibruising, antidepressant, antiemetic, anti-inflammatory, antiseptic, antispasmodic, diaphoretic, digestive, diuretic, laxative, ophthalmic, rubefacient, stimulant

Fir (*Abies Balsamea*)

Analgesic, antibacterial, anti-infectious, anti-inflammatory, antiseptic, antioxidant, aromatic, calming, deodorant, detoxifier, grounding, respiratory, warming

Frankincense (*Boswellia Carteri*)

Analgesic, antiasthmatic, anti-inflammatory, antiseptic, astringent, calming, carminative, cicatrisant, cytophylactic, digestive, disinfectant, diuretic, emenagogue, expectorant, grounding, holy, ritualistic, sedative, spiritual, tonic, uterine, vulnerary

Gardenia (*Gardenia Grandiflora*)

Analgesic, antiabscess, antibacterial, anti-inflammatory, anti-infectious, aphrodisiac, aromatic

Garlic (*Allium Sativum*)

Antibacterial, anticarcinogenic, anticatarrhal, antidandruff, antifungal, antimicrobial, antioxidant, antiseptic, antiviral, carminative, culinary, detoxifier, expectorant, hypotensive, vasodilator

Geranium (*Pelargonium Graveolens*)

Analgesic, antianxiety, antibacterial, antidepressant, antifungal, anti-inflammatory, antiseptic, astringent, bactericidal, cicatrisant, culinary, cytophylactic, deodorant, diuretic, hemostatic, styptic, tonic, vermifuge, vulnerary

Ginger (*Zingiber Officinale*)

Analgesic, antiemetic, anti-inflammatory, antioxidant, antiseptic, antispasmodic, bactericidal, carminative, cephalic, culinary, expectorant, febrifuge, laxative, rubefacient, stimulant, stomachic, sudorific, tonic

Ginkgo Biloba (*Ginkoacea*)

Antiasthmatic, antidepressant, anti-infectious, anti-inflammatory, circulatory, decongestant, energizer, memory booster, nervine

Ginseng (*Panax*)

Antianxiety, anti-inflammatory, antioxidant, aphrodisiac, appetite suppressant, circulatory, immune booster, stimulant, tonic, vasodilator

Grapefruit (*Citrus Paradisii*)

Antianxiety, antidepressant, antioxidant, aperitif, appetite reduction, antiseptic, aromatic, astringent, culinary, disinfectant, diuretic, energizer, lymphatic, stimulant, tonic

Helichrysum/Immortelle (*Helichrysum Angustifolium*)

Analgesic, antiallergenic, antibruising, anticoagulant, antidepressant, antifungal, anti-inflammatory, antimicrobial, antiseptic, antispasmodic, antitussive, cicatrisant, expectorant, hepatic, holy, ritualistic, tonic

Hibiscus (*H Rosa-sinensis*)

Antiallergenic, anticarcinogenic, anticoagulant, antihaematomic, anti-inflammatory, antimicrobial, antiphlogistic, antiseptic, antitussive, aromatic, cholagogue, cicatrisant, cytophylactic, diuretic, dye, emollient, expectorant, febrifuge, fungicidal, hepatic, hypertensive, immune booster, nervine, splenic, weight reduction

Holly (*Llex*)

Antirheumatic, circulation, digestive, hypertensive, protection, purgative

Holy Basil (*Ocimum Sanctum*)

Antibacterial, anti-inflammatory, antioxidant, antiulcer, aromatic, digestive, febrifuge, rituals, spiritual

Honeysuckle (*Lonicera Caprifolium*)

Antibacterial, antifungal, aromatic, culinary, enhances intuition, perfumery

Hyssop (*Hyssopus Officinalis*)

Antiarthritic, antibruising, anti-infectious, antirheumatic, antiseptic, antispasmodic, aromatic, astringent, carminative, cicatrisant, digestive, diuretic, emenagogue, expectorant, febrifuge, holy, hypertensive, nervine, ritualistic, stimulant, sudorific, tonic, vermifuge, vulnerary

Jasmine (*Jasminum Officinale*)

Antianxiety, antidepressant, antiseptic, antispasmodic, aphrodisiac, aromatic, cicatrisant, emenagogue, expectorant, galactogogue, parturient, perfumery, respiratory, rituals, sedative, spiritual, uterine

Juniper Berry (*Juniperus Communis*)

Antifatigue, anti-infectious, anti-inflammatory, antirheumatic, antiseptic, antispasmodic, antitoxic, astringent, carminative, circulatory, energizer, depurative, detoxifying, diuretic, rubefacient, stimulant, stomachic, sudorific, tonic, vulnerary

Lavender (*Lavandula Angustifolia*)

Analgesic, antianxiety, antibiotic, anticonvulsive, antidepressant, antifungal, anti-infectious, anti-inflammatory, antimicrobial, antirheumatic, antiseptic, antispasmodic, antivenous, antiviral, aromatic, bactericidal, calming, cicatrisant, decongestant, deodorant, detoxifying, disinfectant, hypotensive, nervine, perfumery, restorative, sedative, tonic, tranquilizing

- **True Lavender** *(Lavandula Angustifolia)* analgesic, antidepressant, calming, holy, hormonal, rituals, spiritual, vulnerary
- **Spike Lavender** *(Lavandula Latifolia)* analgesic, antiarthritic, aromatic, decongestant, expectorant, insecticidal perfumer, stimulant
- **Lavandin** *(Lavandula X Intermedia)* antidepressant, anti-infectious, calming, cicatrisant, expectorant, nervine, sedative

Lemon (*Citrus Limon*)

Antispasmodic, astringent, aromatic, culinary, detoxifier, germicidal, immune booster, tonic, uplifting

Lemon Balm (*Melissa Officinalis*)

(see Melissa)

Lemongrass (*Cymbopogon Citratus*)

Analgesic, antidepressant, anti-inflammatory, antioxidant, antipyretic, aromatic, astringent, bactericidal, calming, culinary, febrifuge, fungicidal, immune boosting, mood enhancer, nervine, sedative, stomachic, uplifting

Lemon Thyme (*Thymus Citriodorus*)

Antiaging, antianxiety, antiasthmatic, antispasmodic, aromatic, calming, culinary, decongestant, immune boosting, relaxant

Lime (*Citrus Aurantifolia*)

Aperitif, anti-infectious, antiseptic, astringent, antiviral, aperitif, astringent, aromatic, bactericidal, disinfectant, febrifuge, hemostatic, respiratory, restorative, tonic

Linden Blossom (*Flowers*) (*Tilia Cordata*)

Antianxiety, anticarcinogenic, anti-inflammatory, calming, diuretic, expectorant, immune booster, hypertensive

Lotus (*Nelumbo Nucifera*)

Aphrodisiac, aromatic, astringent, calming, chakras, emmenagogue, expectorant, holy, hypotensive, hypnotic, meditative, ritualistic, sedative, tranquilizing, vasodilator, hypnotic

Mandarin (*Citrus Reticulata*)

Antibacterial, antiseptic, antispasmodic, aromatic, antiviral, bactericidal, balancing, calming, circulatory, cytophylactic, depurative, digestive, expectorant, hepatic, nervine, relaxant, sedative, stomachic, tonic

Manuka (*Leptospermum Scoparium*)

Antiallergenic, antianxiety, antibacterial, antidandruff, antifungal, anti-inflammatory, antihistaminic, calming, cicatrisant, cytophylactic, deodorant, nervine, vulnerary

Marjoram (*Origana Majorana*)

Analgesic, aphrodisiac, antiseptic, antispasmodic, antiviral, bactericidal, carminative, cephalic, cordial, diaphoretic, digestive, diuretic, culinary, emenagogue, expectorant, fungicidal, holy, hypotensive, laxative, nervine, ritualistic, sedative, spiritual, stomachic, tranquilizing, vasodilator, vulnerary

Melaleuca (*Melaleuca Quinquenervia*)

(see Tea Tree)

Melissa (Lemon Balm) (*Melissa Officinalis*)

Antibacterial, antidepressant, antihistaminic, antispasmodic, bactericidal, bronchial, carminative, cordial, diaphoretic, emenagogue, febrifuge, hypotensive, insect repellant, nervine, sedative, stomachic, sudorific, tonic, vulnerary

Myrrh (*Balsamodendron Myrrha*)

Analgesic, antibacterial, anticatarrhal, antifungal, anti-inflammatory, antimicrobial, antiseptic, antispasmodic, astringent, carminative, cicatrisant, circulatory, diaphoretic, emollient, expectorant, holy, immune stimulant, mucolytic, revitalizing, rituals, sedative, stimulant, stomachic, tonic, vulnerary

Myrtle (*Myrtus Communis*)

Anti-inflammatory, antimicrobial, antiseptic, astringent, deodorant, digestive, expectorant, nervine, respiratory, sedative, uplifting

Neem (*Azadirachta Indica*)

Antibacterial, anticarcinogenic, antifungal, anti-inflammatory, antioxidant, antiparasitic, antiulcer, antiviral, detoxifier, dental

Neroli (*Citrus Aurantium*)

Antianxiety, antidepressant, anti-infectious, antiseptic, antispasmodic, aphrodisiac, aromatic, bactericidal, carminative, cephalic, cicatrisant, cordial, cytophylactic, deodorant, digestive, disinfectant, emollient, sedative, tonic

Niaouli (*Melaleuca Viridiflora*)

Analgesic, anti-inflammatory, antimalarial, antimicrobial, antirheumatic, antiseptic, bactericidal, balsamic, cicatrisant, decongestant, expectorant, febrifuge, insecticide, respiratory, stimulant, vermifuge, urinary, vulnerary

Orange (*Citrus Cinensis*)

Antibacterial, antidepressant, anti-inflammatory, antimicrobial, aphrodisiac, aromatic, carminative, cholagogue, culinary, immune stimulant, tonic, sedative

Oregano (*Origanum Vulgare*)

Analgesic, antiallergenic, antiarthritic, antibacterial, anticarcinogenic, antifungal, anti-infectious, anti-inflammatory, antioxidant, antiparasitic, antiseptic, antispasmodic, antitoxic, antiviral, bactericidal, culinary, disinfectant, digestive, emenagogue, fungicidal, respiratory, stimulant, tonic

Oregon Grape Root (*Mahonia Aquifolium*)

Antifungal, anti-infectious, antimicrobial, antiulcer, aromatic, cleansing, detoxifying, digestive, skin issues, spiritual

Palmarosa (*Cymbopogon Martinii*)

Antianxiety, antiarthritic, antirheumatic, antiseptic, antiviral, bactericidal, cytophylactic, digestive, febrifuge, hydration balm, nervine, skin issues

Patchouli (*Pogostemon Patchouli*)

Antidepressant, anti-inflammatory, antimicrobial, antiphlogistic, antiseptic, aphrodisiac, aromatic, astringent, bactericidal, calming, cicatrisant, cytophylactic, deodorant, diuretic, emollient, febrifuge, fixative, fungicide, grounding, insecticide, nervine, sedative, tonic

Peppermint (*Mentha Piperita*)

Analgesic, anesthetic, antifungal, anti-infectious, anti-inflammatory, antigalactogogue, antiphlogistic, antiseptic, antispasmodic, aromatic, astringent, carminative, cephalic, cholagogue, cicatrisant, cordial, culinary, decongestant, digestive, emollient, emenagogue, expectorant, febrifuge, hepatic, invigorating, mucolytic, nervine, respiratory, stimulant, stomachic, sudorific, vasoconstrictor, vermifuge, vertigo

Peru Balsam (*Miroxylon Balsamum*)

Antifungal, anti-inflammatory, anti-infectious, antiparasitic, antiseptic, aromatic, calming, grounding, respiratory, vulnerary

Petitgrain (*Citrus Aurantium*)

Antidepressant, antiseptic, antispasmodic, aromatic, balancing, calming, cicatrisant, cosmetic, deodorant, nervine, sedative, uplifting

Pine (*Pinus Sylvestris*)

Analgesic, antibacterial, antioxidant, antirheumatic, antiseptic, aromatic, boosts metabolism, culinary, decongestant, depurative, diuretic, energizing, metabolism, relaxant, rubefacient, urinary

Pink Grapefruit (*Citrus X Paradisi*)

Anticarcinogenic, antioxidant, antiseptic, detoxifier, energizer, purifier, tonic, weight control

Poppy (*Papaver Somniferum*)

Analgesic, anticarcinogenic, antispasmodic, astringent, diaphoretic, expectorant, hypnotic, sedative

Ravensara (*Ravensara Aromatica*)

Analgesic, antiallergenic, antibacterial, antidepressant, anti-inflammatory, antifungal, antimicrobial, antioxidant, antiperspirant, antiseptic, antispasmodic, antitumor, antiviral, aphrodisiac, aromatic, carminative, cicatrisant, disinfectant, diuretic, expectorant, nervine, relaxant, tonic

Roman Chamomile (*Anthermis Nobilis*)

(see Chamomile)

Rose (*Rosa Damascena*)

Antiarthritic, anticarcinogenic, antidepressant, antiphlogistic, antiseptic, antispasmodic, antiviral, aphrodisiac, astringent, aromatic, bactericidal, cholagogue, cicatrisant, culinary, depurative, emenagogue, hemostatic, hepatic, laxative, nervine, stomachic, uterine tonic

Rosemary (*Rosemarinus Officinalis*)

Analgesic, antiaging, antibacterial, anticarcinogenic, anti-inflammatory, antioxidant, antirheumatic, antiseptic, antispasmodic, aromatic, astringent, carminative, circulatory, culinary, decongestant, disinfectant, diuretic, decongestant, digestive, disinfectant, diuretic, immunity booster, memory enhancer, restorative, stimulant, tonic

Sage (*Salvia Officinalis*)

Antiaging, antibacterial, antifungal, anti-inflammatory, antimicrobial, antioxidant, antiseptic, antispasmodic, aromatic, cholagogue, choleretic, cicatrisant, culinary, depurative, digestive, disinfectant, emmenagogue, expectorant, febrifuge, focus, immune booster, laxative, positivity, stimulant

Sandalwood (*Santalum Album*) (Australian Sandalwood—*Santalum Spicatum*)

Antifungal, anti-inflammatory, antiseptic, antiphlogistic, antispasmodic, aphrodisiac, astringent, calming, carminative, cicatrisant, decongestant, disinfectant, diuretic, emollient, expectorant, grounding, harmonizing, hypotensive, insecticide, memory enhancer, mental clarity, relaxing, sedative, tonic

Sesame (*Sesamum Indicum*)

Antiaging, antianxiety, anticarcinogenic, antidepressant, antifungal, anti-inflammatory, antioxidant, antirheumatic, cosmetic, culinary, digestive, grounding, purifying

Spearmint (*Mentha Spicata*)

Antianxiety, antibacterial, antifatigue, antiseptic, antispasmodic, aromatic, calming, carminative, cephalic, circulatory, culinary, emenagogue, expectorant, hormonal, immune boosting, insecticide, nervine, relaxing, restorative, respiratory, stimulant, stomachic tonic

Spikenard (*Nardostachys Jatamansi*)

Antianxiety, antibacterial, antibiotic, antidepressant, antifungal, anti-inflammatory, antioxidant, deodorant, digestive, grounding, holy, laxative, meditative, respiratory, rituals, sedative, spiritual, uterine, vasoconstrictor

Spruce (*Tsuga Canadensis*)

Antiarthritic, anti-infectious, anti-inflammatory, antimicrobial, antirheumatic, antispasmodic, aromatic, disinfectant, expectorant, grounding, immunostimulant, mentally invigorating, respiratory, aromatic, grounding, strengthens nervous system, vulnerary

St. John's Wort (*Hypericum Perforatum*)

Antiarthritic, antianxiety, antidepressant, anti-inflammatory, antineuralgic, antioxidant, antirheumatic, astringent, cicatrisant, cooling, decongestant, hormonal, immunostimulant, vermifuge

Sweet Orange (*Citrus Sinensis*)

Antianxiety, anticarcinogenic, anticoagulant, antidepressant, anti-inflammatory, antimicrobial, antispasmodic, antiseptic, carminative, cholagogue, cicatrisant, circulatory, culinary, detoxifying, digestive, diuretic, energizing, germicidal, relaxing, restorative, stomachic, tonic

Tangerine (*Citrus Reticulata*)

Antibacterial, anticarcinogenic, antifungal, anti-infectious, antiseptic, antispasmodic, antiulcer, aromatic, calming, culinary, cytophylactic, depurative, restorative, sedative, stomachic, tonic, vulnerary weight reduction

Tarragon (*Antemisia Dracunculus*)

Anti-inflammatory, antifatigue, antirheumatic, antiseptic, antispasmodic, aperitif, aromatic, balancing, circulatory, deodorant, detoxifying, digestive, emenagogue, hormonal, stimulant, stomachic vermifuge

Tea Tree (*Melaleuca Alternifolia*)

Antiallergenic, antibacterial, antibiotic, antifungal, anti-infectious, anti-inflammatory, anti-itch, antimicrobial, antiparasitic, antiseptic, antiviral, balsamic, cicatrisant, decongestant, dental, emollient, expectorant, fungicide, immune stimulant, insecticide, respiratory, stimulant, sudorific, vaginal infections, vasodilator, vulnerary

Thyme (*Thymus Vulgaris*)

Antimicrobial, anti-infectious, anti-inflammatory, antirheumatic, antiseptic, antispasmodic, aromatic, bactericidal, bechic, bronchial, cardiac, carminative, cicatrisant, culinary, digestive, diuretic, emenagogue, expectorant, hypertensive, immunostimulant, insecticide, perfumery, restorative, stimulant, tonic, vermifugal

Valerian (*Valeriana Officinalis*)

Analgesic, antianxiety, antidepressant, antispasmodic, calming, cicatrisant, hormonal, nervine, positivity, rituals, sedative, stomachic, tranquilizing

Vanilla (*Vanilla Planifolia*)

Anticarcinogenic, tranquilizing, antidepressant, antioxidant, aphrodisiac, aromatic, culinary, febrifuge, hormonal, relaxing, sedative

Vetiver (*Vetyveria Zizanoides*)

Anticarcinogenic, antidepressant, anti-inflammatory, antioxidant, antiseptic, aphrodisiac, calming, cicatrisant, cooling, febrifuge, relaxant, tranquilizing, sedative

Vitamin E Oil

Antiaging, antiarthritic, antifatigue, anticarcinogenic, antioxidant, antiperspirant, cicatrisant, culinary, emollient, preservative

Wheat Germ (*Triticum Aestivum*)

Antiaging, antioxidant, bactericidal, cell regenerator, emollient

White Fir (*Abies Concolor*)

Analgesic, antiaging, anticarcinogenic, anti-infectious, anti-inflammatory, antioxidant, antirheumatic, antiseptic aromatic, cardiovascular, detoxifying, expectorant, respiratory, rituals, spiritual, weight reduction

Wild Birch (*Betula*)

Antiarthritic, anti-inflammatory, antimucolytic, antineuralgic, antirheumatic, antispasmodic, antitussive, aromatic, astringent, carminative, depurative, diuretic, emenagogue, galactogogue, stimulant, urinary

Wild Orange (*Capparis Mitchellii*)

Antimicrobial, antioxidant, antirheumatic, antiseptic, aromatic, carminative, cicatrisant, cleanser, culinary, depurative, digestive, diuretic, energizer, febrifuge, hypotensive, immune booster, purifying, stomachic, uplifting

Wintergreen (*Gaultheria Procumbens*)

Analgesic, anodyne, antiarthritic, antirheumatic, antispasmodic, antiseptic, aromatic, astringent, calming, carminative, culinary, diuretic, carminative, diuretic, emenagogue, spiritual, stimulant, stress reduction, warming

Yarrow (*Achillea Millefollium*)

Anti-inflammatory, antirheumatic, antiseptic, antispasmodic, astringent, carminative, cicatrisant, circulative, diaphoretic, digestive, expectorant, haemostatic, hypotensive, nervine, stomachic, styptic, tonic, vulnerary

Ylang-Ylang (*Cananga Odorata*)

Antidepressant, anti-infectious, antiseborrhoeic, antiseptic, aphrodisiac, aromatic, balance, calming, cicatrisant, euphoric, hormonal, hypotensive, meditative, nervine, relaxant, sedative, tonic, tranquilizing

References

Alborzian, Cameron. *The One Plan: A Week-by-Week Guide to Restoring Your Natural Health and Happiness*. New York: HarperOne, 2013.

Amazing-Solutions. "20 Popular Aromatherapy Oils (And When to Use Them)." Accessed 2017.
https://amazing-solutions.com/article/popular-aromatherapy-oils/.

Amrita. "Essential Oils Uses Chart." Accessed 2016.
www.amrita.net/essential-oils-chart.

AromaWeb. "Tea Tree Oil." Accessed December 6, 2015.
https://www.aromaweb.com/essential-oils/tea-tree-oil.asp

Axe, Dr. Josh. "101 Essential Oil Uses and Benefits." Accessed August 2, 2017.
draxe.com/essential-oil-uses-benefits/.

Axe, Dr. Josh, and Eric Zielinski. "Top 25 Peppermint Oil Uses and Benefits." Accessed August 17, 2017. draxe.com/peppermint-oil-uses-benefits/.

Bible, Holman. *Holy Bible: Holman Christian Standard, Ultrathin Reference Bible, Teal Leathertouch*. Holman Bible Pub, 2016.

Bremness, Lesley. *Herbs*. New York: Dorling Kindersley, 1994.

Bretherton, Linda, and Jim Whitham. *Dosha for Life: A Contemporary Examination of the Ancient Ayurvedic Science of Self-Healing.* Findhorn, Scotland: Findhorn Press, 2007.

Bulk Apothecary Supplier. "Essential Oils." Accessed January 11, 2016. www.bulkapothecary.com/categories/essential-oils/pure-therapeutic-grade/.

Dodt, Colleen K. *The Essential Oils Book: Creating Personal Blends for Mind & Body.* Pownal, VT: Storey Communications, 1996.

Eden's Garden. "150 Ways To Use Essential Oils." Accessed December 16, 2016. www.edensgarden.com/pages/home.

Fite, Vannoy Gentles, Michele McDaniel Gentles, and Vannoy Reynolds Lin. *Essential Oils for Healing: Over 400 All-Natural Recipes for Everyday Ailments.* New York: Macmillan, 2016.

Frawley, David. *Ayurveda, Nature's Medicine.* Twin Lakes, WI: Lotus, 2001.

———*Ayurveda and the Mind: the Healing of Consciousness.* Twin Lakes, WI: Lotus, 1997.

———*Ayurvedic Healing: A Comprehensive Guide.* Twin Lakes, WI: Lotus, 2000.

Group, Dr. Edward, DC, NP, DACBN, DCBCN, DABFM. "Best Essential Oils and Their Benefits." Accessed December 1, 2016. www.globalhealingcenter.com/natural-health/best-essential-oils-and-their-benefits/.

Healthy Traditions. "Essential Oils." Accessed August 2, 2016. healthytraditions.com/healthytraditions/essential-oils.html.

Herbal Supplement Resource. "Bay Laurel Benefits, Side Effects and Uses." Accessed August 20, 2017. www.herbal-supplement-resource.com/bay-laurel-benefits.html.

Herbwisdom. "A-Z Herb List." Accessed August 4, 2016. https://www.herbwisdom.com/herblist.html.

———"Herb Information, Benefits, Discussion and News." Accessed April 2, 2015. www.herbwisdom.com/herbinformation.

Higley, Connie, et al. *Aromatherapy A-Z.* Carlsbad, CA: Hay House, 2002.

Judith, Anodea, and Selene Vega. *The Sevenfold Journey: Reclaiming Mind, Body & Spirit through the Chakras.* Freedom, CA: Crossing, 1993.

Keville, Kathi, and Mindy Green. *Aromatherapy: A Complete Guide to the Healing Art.* Berkeley, CA: Crossing Press, 2009.

Kowalchik, Claire, William Hylton H., and Anna Carr. *Rodale's Illustrated Encyclopedia of Herbs.* Emmaus, PA: Rodale, 1987.

Lad, Vasant. *The Complete Book of Ayurvedic Home Remedies.* New York: Harmony, 1998.

Lad, Vasant, and David Frawley. *The Yoga of Herbs: An Ayurvedic Guide to Herbal Medicine.* Santa Fe, NM: Lotus, 1986.

Lavabre, Marcel F. *Aromatherapy Workbook.* Rochester, VT: Healing Arts Press, 1997.

Mama, Katie. "Risks and Uses of Essential Oils." Wellness Mama. Accessed August 28, 2017. wellnessmama.com/26519/essential-oils-risks/.

Mountain Rose Herbs. "Organic Herbs & Spices." Accessed July 22, 2016. www.mountainroseherbs.com/aromatherapy.

N., Anthony. "Essential Oils and Aromatherapy: Beginner's Guide to Using Essential Oils." *Essential Oils Beginner's Guide: Complete Uses & Benefits,* Accessed May 20, 2017. www.swansonvitamins.com/blog/natural-health-tips/essential-oils-aromatherapy-guide.

National Association for Holistic Aromatherapy. "Exploring Aromatherapy." Accessed May 29, 2016. naha.org.

Natural News. "Use peppermint oil to aid digestion, repel bugs, and more." Accessed 2016. www.naturalnews.com/042219_peppermint_healing_herbs_digestion.html.

New Directions Aromatics. "About Essential Oils: Everything You Need To Know About Essential Oils." Accessed March 13, 2017. www.newdirectionsaromatics.com/blog/products/about-essential-oils.html.

Organic Facts. "List of Essential Oils." Accessed March 30, 2015. www.organicfacts.net/health-benefits/essential-oils.

Price, Shirley. *The Aromatherapy Workbook: Understanding Essential Oils from Plant to User.* London: Thorsons, 2000.

Spear, Heidi E. *The Everything Guide to Chakra Healing.* Avons, MA: Adams Media Corporation, 2012.

Spirit Science. "Ancient Oils: 3 Ways the Egyptians Used Essential Oils." Accessed April 20, 2017.
thespiritscience.net/2016/08/21/ancient-oils-3-ways-the-egyptians-used-essential-oils/.

Sustainable Baby Steps. "An Introductory Guide to 1000's of Uses for Essential Oils." Accessed June 10, 2016.
www.sustainablebabysteps.com/uses-for-essential-oils.html.

Tirtha, Sada Shiva. *The Ayurveda Encyclopedia: Natural Secrets to Healing, Prevention & Longevity*. Bayville, NY: Ayurveda Holistic Center, 1998.

University of Minnesota. "Are Essential Oils Safe?" Accessed June 2, 2016.
www.takingcharge.csh.umn.edu/explore-healing-practices/aromatherapy/are-essential-oils-safe.

Worwood, Susan E., and Valerie Ann Worwood. *Essential Aromatherapy: A Pocket Guide to Essential Oils and Aromatherapy*. Novato, CA: New World Library, 2003.

Z, Dr. Eric. "10 Best Essential Oils for Healing and How to Use Them!" Accessed June 23, 2017. drericz.com/best-essential-oils/.

Websites

anniesremedy.com

aromatherapybible.com

aromatics.com

blog-ovviooils.com

essentialoils.com

healthybenefits.com

livestrong.com

mercola.com

naturesgift.com

organicfacts.com

usingeossafely.com

webmd.com

wellnessmama.com

Index

To Write to the Author

If you wish to contact the author or would like more information about this book, please write to the author in care of Llewellyn Worldwide Ltd. and we will forward your request. Both the author and publisher appreciate hearing from you and learning of your enjoyment of this book and how it has helped you. Llewellyn Worldwide Ltd. cannot guarantee that every letter written to the author can be answered, but all will be forwarded. Please write to:

Vannoy Gentles Fite
℅ Llewellyn Worldwide
2143 Wooddale Drive
Woodbury, MN 55125-2989

Please enclose a self-addressed stamped envelope for reply,
or $1.00 to cover costs. If outside the U.S.A., enclose
an international postal reply coupon.

Many of Llewellyn's authors have websites with additional information and resources. For more information, please visit our website at

http://www.llewellyn.com